Solving Back Problems

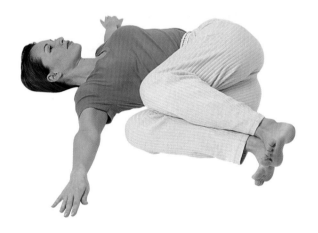

Jenny Sutcliffe, M.D.

TIME
LIFE
BOOKS
Alexandria, Virginia

Time-Life Books is a division of Time Life Inc.

TIME LIFE INC.

PRESIDENT AND CEO: George Artandi

TIME-LIFE CUSTOM PUBLISHING

Vice President and Publisher	Terry Newell
Vice President of Sales and Marketing	Neil Levin
Director of Acquisitions and Editorial Resources	Jennifer Pearce
Director of Creative Services	Laura Ciccone McNeill
Director of Special Markets	Liz Ziehl
Project Manager	Jennie Halfant

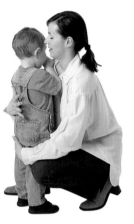

First printing. Printed in China

TIME-LIFE is a trademark of Time Warner Inc. U.S.A.

Library of Congress Cataloging-in-Publication Data

Sutcliffe, Jenny.
    Solving back problems / Jenny Sutcliffe.
        p. cm. -- (Time-Life health factfiles)
    Includes index.
    ISBN 0-7370-1607-8 (pbk.)
    1. Backache--Prevention. I. Title. II. Series.
RD768.S82 1999
617.5'64--dc21   99-26902
                                                        CIP

Books produced by Time-Life Custom Publishing are available at a
special bulk discount for promotional and premium use. Custom
adaptations can also be created to meet your specific marketing
goals. Call 1-800-323-5255.

A Marshall Edition
Conceived, edited and designed by
Marshall Editions
161 New Bond Street
London W1Y 9PA

Note

Every effort has been taken to
ensure that all information in
this book is correct and
compatible with national
standards generally accepted at
the time of publication. This
book is not intended to replace
consultation with your doctor
or other healthcare
professional. The author and
publisher disclaim any liability,
loss, injury, or damage
incurred as a consequence,
directly or indirectly, of the
use and application of the
contents of this book.

CONTENTS

Preventing Back Problems

Special Conditions

Professional Help

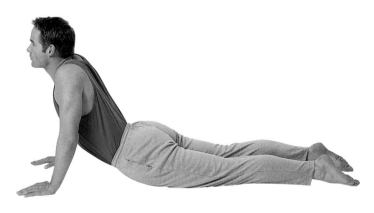

INTRODUCTION

When the ancestors of the human race first started to walk upright on two legs, hundreds of thousands of years ago, it was a turning point in our evolution and one that helped to define our preeminence in the animal kingdom. However, in terms of the evolution of our bodies at least, we were ill-prepared to take such a giant step forward. For the fact is that though the human back is a superb piece of precision engineering, it is not yet fully adapted to coping with the demands of walking upright – in evolutionary terms, it was only yesterday that we started to do so. As a result, the human back is extremely vulnerable to damage – in fact, if you take colds and flu out of the equation, back pain is the most common cause of absence from work in industrialized countries. And even when back pain is not serious enough to make it impossible to work, it is still a perennial, nagging problem, and something that reduces the quality of life for millions of people.

THE SOLUTION

This book is designed to help prevent back problems from occurring and, when something does go wrong, help to solve the pain, discomfort, and feelings of helplessness by which back problems are characterized. It begins by telling you how to prevent the basic structural limitations of the human body from affecting your life in the first place, and to show you what to do if you already have back problems or develop them. More importantly, though, it takes into account the fact that there has been a considerable change in the way that the medical profession approaches the treatment of back problems over the last few decades. At one time, people suffering from back pain or injuries were advised to rest, immobile, in bed for day after day. But now research has shown that immobility is not the answer. Instead, the emphasis is now on regaining mobility as soon as possible by means of a series of carefully graded exercises – as this book shows you.

UNDERSTANDING YOUR BACK

If you know how your back works and understand the limitations and vulnerabilities that are imposed on it by its design, you are halfway to coming to terms with preventing a back problem from developing. So, Chapter 1 tells you how your back works: you will discover the detail of how the intricate system of checks and balances in the anatomy of the spine, its joints, and its supporting muscles and ligaments works and what makes it prone to failure.

AN ATTACK OF BACK PAIN

The action you take when you first experience a back problem is of critical importance in determining how quickly you recover. Chapter 2 advises you on what to do when you have an acute – sudden – attack of back pain, with information on what to do first to prevent making the problem worse, when to see your doctor and a detailed prescription of gentle exercises and rest positions that can help alleviate the problem.

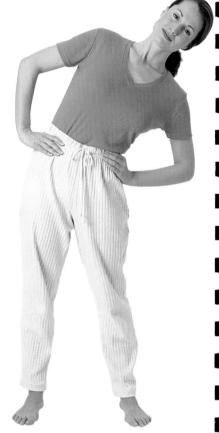

LIVING WITH LONG-TERM BACK PROBLEMS

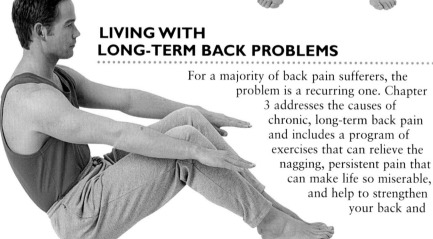

For a majority of back pain sufferers, the problem is a recurring one. Chapter 3 addresses the causes of chronic, long-term back pain and includes a program of exercises that can relieve the nagging, persistent pain that can make life so miserable, and help to strengthen your back and abdomen to protect against further attacks of pain. The chapter also includes practical tips and strategies for avoiding chronic back problems.

PRESERVING BACK HEALTH

Because of the inherent vulnerability of the spine to injury and strain, we are all potential back-pain sufferers. For this reason, everyone can benefit from the advice on preventing back trouble given in Chapter 4. Here you will find out how you can avoid injuring your back or aggravating a pre-existing condition and so vastly improve your quality of life at all ages: you will discover how to correct your posture, for example, and so reduce the stresses on your back; how to lift correctly; how to adjust your working environment for maximum safety and minimum risk; how to make driving a risk-free experience, in terms of your back, at least; and so on.

SPECIAL CAUSES OF BACK PAIN

Not all back pain is simply the result of injury or strain. In some cases, particular medical problems underlie acute or chronic back problems. Chapter 5 describes some of these conditions and provides specific advice, for example, on the problems of osteoarthritis and osteoporosis, the scourge of postmenopausal women – and how to avoid them. The special stresses placed on the back by pregnancy and the body's natural aging processes are also discussed.

PROFESSIONAL HELP

Finally, Chapter 6 is devoted to the types of professional help available, including physical therapy and a variety of alternative therapies, and offers advice on how to go about getting such help. For it must be stressed that this book is a guide only and that nothing can substitute for individual medical advice and treatment that is prescribed specifically for you. If you are in any doubt whatsoever about your condition, or if your back pain is either extremely severe or has persisted for longer than 48 hours, you should consult your doctor without delay.

A PAIN-FREE LIFE

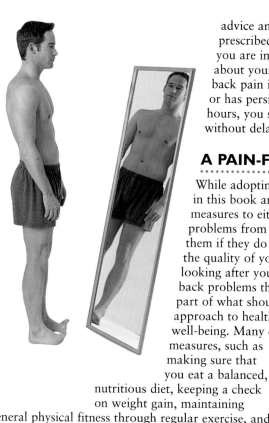

While adopting the strategies contained in this book and taking proactive measures to either prevent back problems from developing or treating them if they do occur will help improve the quality of your life enormously, looking after your back and treating any back problems that develop is only one part of what should be an overall strategic approach to health and your personal well-being. Many commonsense health measures, such as making sure that you eat a balanced, nutritious diet, keeping a check on weight gain, maintaining general physical fitness through regular exercise, and utilizing effective stress reduction and relaxation-enhancing measures, play an important part in ensuring that you do not experience back problems. The back can benefit enormously from a holistic approach to medicine and health. So the message is follow the exercise regimes described in this book, but remember, too, to examine your entire lifestyle if you want to definitively lower your risk of developing a back trouble or having an existing problem recur.

THE STRUCTURE OF THE BACK

1

The human back comprises a complex arrangement of living tissues. It is nourished by a rich blood supply and protects the body's most important nerve pathways. The bones and cartilage of the spine form a column of joints that are held in place by a network of ligaments, muscles, and tendons designed to maximize both strength and flexibility. Considered purely in engineering terms, the arrangement is very sophisticated and precise – but it is these very qualities that make the back vulnerable to stresses and strains and wear and tear. This section of the book describes how the various elements of the back function and looks at how pain is transmitted in different ways through its pathways.

STRUCTURE OF THE SPINE

The spinal column is a marvelous piece of engineering that performs a range of functions and endures a wide variety of stresses and strains. It is made up of 34 bones called vertebrae that are stacked on top of each other and separated by cartilaginous pads, or disks. The column is held together by strong ligaments and by the facet joints between the vertebrae. The result is a structure that has both great strength and considerable flexibility. Despite this, the demands that daily living place on the spine make it the most vulnerable part of the skeleton, and it is, as a result, a common site for aches and pains.

FUNCTIONS OF THE SPINE

- To support the head and give rigidity to the skeleton.

- To maintain an upright posture.

- To protect the spinal cord, which carries nerves between the brain and the rest of the body.

- To give attachments for muscles and ribs.

- To act as a shock absorber.

- To allow the body to perform a wide range of movements.

REGIONS OF THE SPINE

- The seven cervical vertebrae at the neck support and balance the head. Two specialized vertebrae at the base of the skull, the atlas and the axis, act rather like a universal joint, allowing the head to rotate and move backward and forward.

- The twelve thoracic vertebrae are connected to the ribs, together forming the ribcage. The ribcage allows enough movement for the lungs to expand during breathing and protects many vital organs.

- The five lumbar vertebrae form the lower back, or the "small of the back." They connect to the sacrum at the top of the buttocks.

- The sacrum comprises five bones fused together and forms, with the pelvis, a bony basin to protect the bladder and reproductive organs.

- The coccyx at the base of the spine is our vestigial tail. It is made up of four bones fused together and has no function in humans.

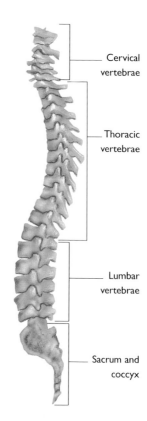

Cervical vertebrae

Thoracic vertebrae

Lumbar vertebrae

Sacrum and coccyx

THE CURVES OF THE SPINE

The back is not straight – nor should it be – as it is the curves in the spine that give it the ability to absorb the stresses of maintaining an upright posture. The thoracic and sacral vertebrae curve backward and are known as primary curves because they are present at birth. The cervical and lumbar vertebrae curve forward. The cervical curve develops as the baby learns to lift its head, and the lumbar curve develops as the baby learns to sit. Viewed from the side, the cervical and lumbar curves are concave and the thoracic and sacral curves convex.

NATURALLY SPRUNG

These natural curves act like a spring to give the spine resilience to the forces of gravity and to the shock waves from the ground as we walk or run. If the back is habitually held too straight or over-curved, the spinal column and its muscles and ligaments cannot absorb the everyday shocks and stresses and will start to malfunction. The muscles and ligaments will either be over-stretched or too taut, and the bones and joints of the spine will be liable to wear and tear – the result being backache.

EXCESSIVE CURVES

Medically, an exaggerated convex curve is called kyphosis and an exaggerated concave curve is known as lordosis. If all the curves are exaggerated the condition is known as kypho-lordosis. Occasionally, a spine will curve to the side in an S or C shape. This defect, known as scoliosis, is usually present at birth, but it can also sometimes be a postural defect caused by increased tension in the muscles on one side of the spine. For more detail on these problems, see pages 100-101.

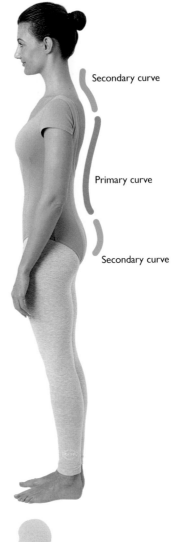

Secondary curve

Primary curve

Secondary curve

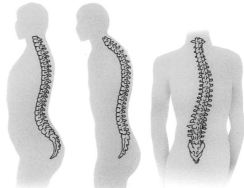

Kyphosis   Lordosis   Scoliosis

JOINTS AND LIGAMENTS

The bones in the body are living things that have a rich blood and nerve supply and a continuous and rapid turnover of nutrients – in particular, the minerals calcium and phosphorus and vitamin D. Bone marrow found within the larger bones is the site for the manufacture of the blood cells that are vital to the immune system and the transport of oxygen around the body. The bones are held together by joints, strengthened by ligaments, to form the skeleton that supports and protects the soft tissues of the body and allows us to move.

THE STRUCTURE OF THE VERTEBRAE

A typical vertebra is composed of five parts:

■ The main part, or body, is composed of cancellous bone surrounded by a layer of compact bone. Compact bone resembles ivory and is very strong and solid. Cancellous bone is spongy and springy and is composed of large numbers of interwoven bony fibers. These fibers are what give the bone its ability to absorb and transmit pressure. As the weight of the body is transmitted down the spine to the hips, and finally the ground, the vertebrae get progressively larger in order to be able to cope with the increasing pressure.

■ The neural or vertebral arch is a strong arch of bone that protects the spinal cord as it passes down from the brain to the lumbar spine.

■ The three vertebral processes are bony projections from the vertebral body. The transverse processes, on each side, and the spinous process, which you can feel at the back of the spine, provide points of contact for muscles and ligaments.

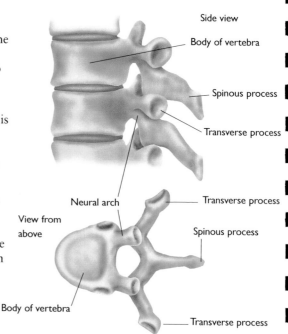

Side view

Body of vertebra

Spinous process

Transverse process

Neural arch

Transverse process

View from above

Spinous process

Body of vertebra

Transverse process

THE FACET JOINTS

Each vertebra also has four facet surfaces – on the upper and lower surfaces of the two transverse processes – that articulate with the vertebrae above and below. For more information about these important joints, see page 43.

INTERVERTEBRAL DISKS

The vertebrae are separated and cushioned from each other by pads of cartilaginous material known as intervertebral disks. These act as shock absorbers and allow for compression and distortion along the spinal column. The disks are rather like flattened hard candy with gooey centers. The center of the disk is filled with a jelly-like substance that is 85 percent water and is called the *nucleus pulposus*. This is surrounded by tough elastic fibers that are interwoven into rings, known as *annular fibrosa*. The disks allow movement by molding themselves into the space available like a balloon full of water.

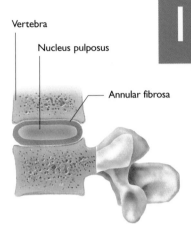

Vertebra

Nucleus pulposus

Annular fibrosa

WHAT IS A SLIPPED DISK?

Standing, lifting, and other daily activities put great pressure on the disks, and they may bulge out or into the body of the vertebra. The disk usually returns to its normal shape during rest or sleep. However, if subjected to extreme pressure, the *nucleus pulposus* may break through its covering; when this puts pressure on a nerve, the result is the painful condition known as a "slipped" (or prolapsed) disk.

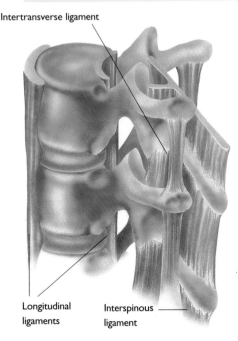

Intertransverse ligament

Longitudinal ligaments

Interspinous ligament

LIGAMENTS

A ligament is a strong band of fibrous tissue that runs from one bone to another, to protect and reinforce a joint. Ligaments have some "give" but, depending on their length, will limit or prevent movement in one or more directions. The main ligaments of the spine, the longitudinal ligaments, run the whole length from top to bottom in front, behind, and to the sides of the vertebral bodies. Others connect the individual vertebrae, running from process to process, and surrounding the facet joints. Ligaments that are not moved enough become stiff; those that are overstretched for long periods become lax. The first will limit movement, and the second will allow too much.

MUSCLES AND THE SPINE

Each muscle consists of millions of long fibers, bound into bundles by connective tissue. Each individual muscle contains many of these bundles wrapped in an outer sheath, all richly supplied with blood and nerves. Muscle tissue is designed to contract and relax. Skeletal muscles are attached at each end to a bone by a tendon: a fibrous cord covered by a lubricated sheath that allows it to glide over other tendons or bones. When a muscle contracts, it pulls on the bones and produces movement. It also maintains posture and produces body heat. Muscles tend to work in opposing pairs – when one contracts the other relaxes.

BACK MUSCLES

The muscles of the back are arranged in several layers, and no muscle crosses the midline – the spine. Instead, each muscle has a matching muscle on the other side.

■ The deepest muscles are short and dense, extending only from one vertebra to the next. As long as the muscles on each side are of equal strength, they keep the vertebrae in alignment and the spine stays stable and upright.

■ The muscles of the next layer are strap-shaped and originate mainly from the pelvis, from where they fan out and attach themselves to various vertebrae, ribs, and even the head. They are mostly concerned with fine adjustment and control of the large back muscles that control posture.

■ The largest back muscles form the outer layer and are mainly broad triangular sheets of muscle that join the spinal processes of the vertebrae to the shoulder blades and shoulder joints. These are powerful postural muscles and keep the trunk stable when you use your arms, especially when lifting. The muscle that contracts to pull the body upright is in this layer.

ABDOMINAL MUSCLES

The abdominal muscles act as a counter to the back muscles by exerting a forward pull to balance the backward pull of the back muscles. They contract to allow the spine to bend by pulling the ribcage closer to the pelvis.

■ The loin muscle, or *psoas*, is a deep abdominal muscle that is joined to the lumbar vertebrae, passes over the front of the hip joint, and ends on the thigh bone. The *psoas* compresses the lumbar disks when it contracts, as in sitting up from a lying position.

■ The other large abdominal muscles have an indirect effect on the spine. When they are contracted, they increase the pressure inside the abdominal cavity so it can absorb some of the pressure from the spine. If the abdominals are slack, any pressure, especially during lifting, is borne primarily by the spine and the back muscles.

RANGE OF MOVEMENT

The vertebral column can move in a number of directions on a vertical plane.
The greatest degree of movement is allowed in the forward bend.

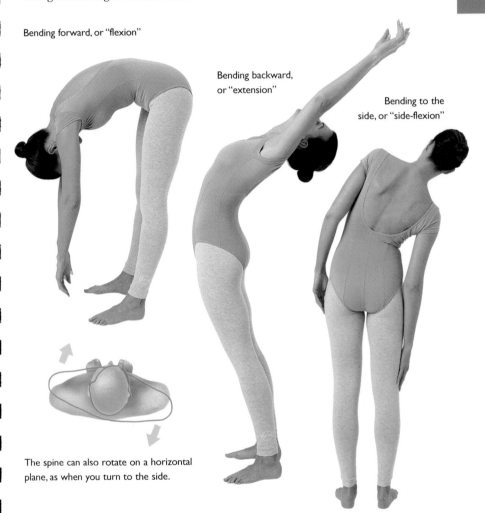

Bending forward, or "flexion"

Bending backward,
or "extension"

Bending to the
side, or "side-flexion"

The spine can also rotate on a horizontal
plane, as when you turn to the side.

WHERE THE MOVEMENTS OCCUR

There is a greater range of movement in the cervical and lumbar regions than
the thoracic. This is due to the ratio between the thickness of the vertebrae
and the disks, and to the tension of the ligaments. However, the majority of
rotation occurs in the thoracic spine. The lumbar spine allows 80 percent of
the movement of forward flexion, which is why it is so vulnerable to strains.
Twenty percent of the movement occurs between the fourth and fifth vertebrae
and 60 percent between the fifth lumbar vertebra and the first sacral vertebra.

THE SPINAL CORD

One of the essential functions of the spine is to protect the spinal cord. This connects the brain to the peripheral nervous system, carrying sensory information from the body to the brain and returning the brain's instructions to the muscles for action. Any damage to the spine that involves the nerves of the spinal cord or its branches can cause pain or even paralysis in almost any part of the body. Sciatica, for example, is caused by the pinching of the sciatic nerve where it leaves the lumbar vertebrae, often due to a ruptured intervertebral disk. The potentially drastic consequences of spinal cord damage provide a powerful argument for taking care of your back.

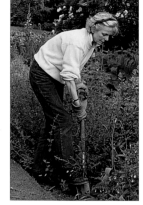

Strain from digging is a common cause of sciatica.

ANATOMY OF THE SPINAL CORD

The spinal cord is a part of the central nervous system. It runs for about 18 inches from the base of the brain to the lumbar vertebrae, where the remaining nerves branch out. This bottom part is known as the *cauda equina*, which is Latin for "horse's tail."

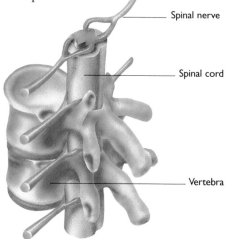

Spinal nerve

Spinal cord

Vertebra

■ The cord is cylindrical in shape and is composed of blood vessels and an inner core of nerve fibers. At regular intervals, spinal nerves branch off the cord and pass through gaps between the facet joints and the main vertebral body. These then divide to form a network of smaller branches, each supplying a particular area of the body.

■ The spinal cord runs down and is protected by the bony tube formed by the vertebrae and the small spinal ligaments and muscles. It is bathed in cerebrospinal fluid, which is retained by three concentric tubes known collectively as the dura. The fluid acts as a shock absorber to protect the spinal column from pressure.

■ The whole cord can stretch to adapt to changing positions and is difficult to damage unless the spine dislocates or is fractured, or something sharp pierces the cord.

SPINAL NERVES

The spinal nerves are made up of millions of individual nerve fibers or neurons. They fall into three categories:

■ Motor, or "efferent," nerves that control the movements of muscles.

■ Sensory, or "afferent," nerves that carry impulses from the sensory nerve endings in the body to the spinal column and brain.

■ Mixed nerves that consist of both motor and sensory nerves. The spinal nerves are all mixed nerves carrying sensory information up to the brain and motor information down from it. Each spinal nerve covers a specific area of the body so it is possible to relate different spinal nerves to different areas of the body with some accuracy.

■ Nerves from the neck, or cervical, region supply the arms and shoulders.

■ Nerves from the thoracic region supply the trunk.

■ Nerves from the lumbar and sacral regions supply the buttocks and legs.

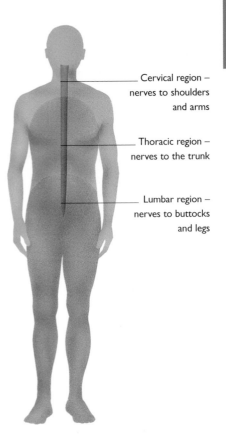

Cervical region – nerves to shoulders and arms

Thoracic region – nerves to the trunk

Lumbar region – nerves to buttocks and legs

The area of skin supplied by a particular spinal nerve is called a dermatome. On the trunk these form a series of regular segments running around the body. In the limbs the situation is more complicated since two spinal nerves may supply a single area. Nevertheless, numbness or pain over a particular skin area will give a therapist a good idea which nerve root is affected in a spinal problem. For example, numbness or pain over the shoulder indicates pressure on the spinal nerve arising between cervical vertebrae three and four.

Warning

If you find someone who has been involved in an accident or otherwise injured and you suspect that their spine may have been damaged, do not attempt to move them unless the situation is life-threatening. Summon medical assistance immediately. Damage to the spinal cord through the application of incorrect handling techniques may have serious long-term neurological consequences.

HOW WE FEEL PAIN

Pain is the body's alarm signal. It tells the brain that something is wrong and allows appropriate action to be taken. Unpleasant though it is, pain is vital for survival. It alerts us to the threat of physical injury and warns us of diseases and other problems of which we might otherwise have been unaware. Pain is generated in the brain in response to signals from specialized pain receptors in the skin, organs, and other tissues. Those in the skin are mainly responsible for the detection of external threats, such as fire or wounds, while those in the deeper tissues mainly respond to internal injury and disease.

TYPES OF PAIN

There are two types of pain, each of which serves a different function in terms of the warning it sends to the brain. These are acute pain and chronic pain.

Category of pain	Features and purpose	Examples
Acute pain	Sharp, intense pain. Serves to warn of an immediate and potentially serious threat to the body.	Injury, such as a cut or burn.
Chronic pain	Persistent dull aching, or soreness and tenderness in the affected area. Serves to warn that some form of damage is occurring, or has already occurred.	Can accompany malfunction or disease in part of the body. Headaches and backaches are examples.

PAIN FIBERS

Acute and chronic pain also differ in the way they travel to and from the brain. Different types of nerve fibers are involved. Acute pain travels along A-fibers. These are surrounded by a myelin sheath – a type of fatty insulating material. As a result, nerve impulses travel along them at great speed – about 30 feet per second. Chronic pain travels along C-fibers. These have no insulating myelin sheath, and nerve impulses travel at much lower speeds – about 3 feet per second, or ten times slower than those carried by the A-fibers. C-fibers are usually found deep in the tissues.

PAIN THRESHOLDS

Pain receptors work on an "all or nothing" system. When they are stimulated beyond a certain threshold, they send a message of pain; if the stimulation fails to reach the threshold, they do not. Pain varies in intensity not because the signals are stronger or weaker but because of differences in the number and frequency of messages the brain receives. And even when a pain signal has been activated, it may not reach the brain – there are three junctions, or "gates," between the pain receptors and the brain's sensory cortex to which the sensation of pain is directed.

GATEWAYS

The first junction is in the spinal cord, and it operates on the principle known as the "gateway theory." According to this, the gate can only take a limited amount of traffic. If too many signals try to get through the gate, priority is given to the fast A-fibers: signals traveling along the slower C-fibers simply cannot get through. Once the first flood of acute pain impulses has died down, the messages carried by the C-fibers are allowed to pass through again. The other gates, in the brain, operate on a different principle. These gates use the body's own natural painkillers, called endorphins, to reduce or block the pain (see page 20).

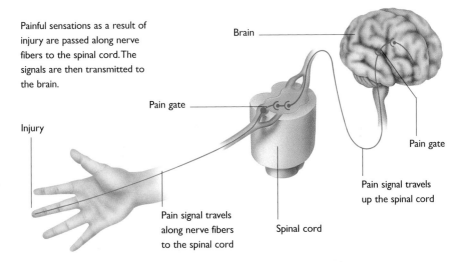

Painful sensations as a result of injury are passed along nerve fibers to the spinal cord. The signals are then transmitted to the brain.

Brain

Pain gate

Injury

Pain gate

Pain signal travels up the spinal cord

Pain signal travels along nerve fibers to the spinal cord

Spinal cord

RUBBING IT BETTER

Pressure sensations travel to the brain along the same type of nerve fibers as acute pain – the fast A-fibers. This gives them priority over the slower signals of chronic pain, which are therefore blocked or much reduced at the gateway in the spine. This is why rubbing a hurt better really does work.

NATURAL PAINKILLERS

Endorphins are chemicals that closely resemble the "transmitter" substances that carry nerve impulses from one nerve fiber to another. The release of these chemicals in the brain and nervous system can block the sensation of pain and promote a sense of well-being. Hence, they are often known as the body's natural painkillers.

BIOCHEMICAL PAIN BARRIERS

The nervous pathways from sensory receptors to the brain are not composed of single nerve fibers: there are several links in the chain. At a junction, the impulse must be communicated between nerve fibers, and this is the function of the transmitter molecules. Endorphins mimic the characteristics of the transmitter molecules, occupying the receptor sites on the nerve fibers that would normally receive the pain signal, but without carrying the impulses forward. As a result, they block pain signals from reaching the brain. There are varying amounts of endorphins in the body, but there are several things that can stimulate production:

- Exercise – endorphins produce the "runner's high."

- Deep relaxation.

- Contentment.

- Sleep.

- A positive mental outlook.

FIGHT OR FLIGHT

Endorphins are also released as part of the "fight or flight" response (see pages 84-85). This is why people may not realize they have been hurt when they are involved in a traumatic event – the pain is kept at bay until the incident is over.

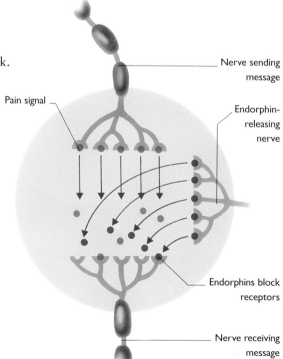

Nerve sending message

Pain signal

Endorphin-releasing nerve

Endorphins block receptors

Nerve receiving message

ACUTE BACK PAIN

A sudden attack of acute back pain can be very debilitating and distressing, but it is not necessarily a sign that you will always have a "bad back." More often than not, it is a response to a chronic problem, but once the acute pain has been relieved and the muscles, ligaments, and joints of the back have been returned to a less critical condition, the chronic problem can be addressed. The key to treatment of acute back pain is a phased program of exercise and rest. In this section you will find out what to do in response to an attack and when to call the doctor, and be taken through a staged recovery program with exercises, rest positions, and self-help measures.

WHAT ARE THE CAUSES?

The most common causes of acute back pain are a chronic, long-term back problem, such as poor posture or weakness of the abdominal muscles. These faults can increase the stresses and strains on the spine and the spinal muscles to such an extent that damage results. Degenerative conditions, such as osteoarthritis or osteoporosis, may also cause acute back pain if they have progressed to such an extent that the tissues have been damaged. In such cases there may be temporary relief after a day or so, but it is likely that episodes of acute pain will recur unless the underlying chronic problem is resolved.

CHRONIC CAUSES OF ACUTE BACK PAIN

When an attack of acute back pain is the result of damage caused by a chronic condition, the most likely causes are:

- Incorrect posture (see pages 68-71).
- Weak abdominal muscles (see pages 80-81).
- Osteoarthritis (see pages 94-95).
- Osteoporosis (see pages 96-97).

MECHANICAL CAUSES OF ACUTE PAIN

A chronic condition is by no means always at the root of acute back pain, however. An attack can often be triggered by a movement that seems minor in itself, such as bending over to pick up a handbag from the floor, but the real damage has usually been done a day or so earlier during any unaccustomed physical exertion. At such times it is easy for muscles to become over-tense and strained as they attempt to protect the back from the unusual demands being made on it; unusual strain may also be put on ligaments and the vertebrae and intervertebral disks.

By the next day, the muscles may either be stiff and aching or have relaxed to such an extent that they no longer support the spine adequately, while the ligaments and joints have not yet returned to the state they were in before the exercise. This purely mechanical damage destabilizes the whole system, with the result that a seemingly harmless movement can prove to be the last straw, causing muscle spasms, pulled ligaments, protrusion of an intervertebral disk, or inflammation of the facet joints. Incorrect lifting and strain from unaccustomed exercise are typical causes.

INCORRECT LIFTING

Incorrect lifting
technique – for example,
when leaning forward to
lift heavy baggage out of
the trunk of a car – can
easily strain your back.
Lifting with a bent back
doubles the compression
pressure on the
intervertebral joints,
with the result that a
joint, ligament, or disk
that is already weak is
unable to cope with the
extra stress.

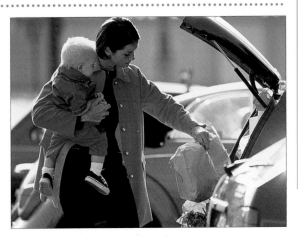

EXCESSIVE OR UNACCUSTOMED EXERCISE

Strenuous exercise, especially if it involves twisting – as, for example, in a game
of racquetball, or dancing, is a common cause of acute back pain. In some
forms of exercise the movements are predominantly in one direction: bending
forward, or flexion, and use only one set of muscles. The opposite muscles –
those that extend the spine, stretching it out – become over-stretched, weak,
and unable to contract fully farther than the upright mid-position. This means
that the muscles and ligaments are not strong enough or flexible enough to
withstand the increased pressure when a twisting movement is made.

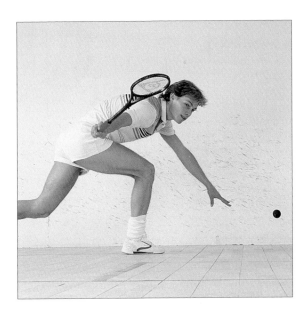

Warning

Urgent medical
attention is required if
any accident or fall
involves part of the
spine. The victim
should not be moved
at all, unless under
medical supervision,
until the spine has
been X-rayed to
eliminate a dislocation
or fracture of the
spinal column.

WHAT SHOULD I DO?

When acute pain strikes, first, stop whatever it is that you are doing and lie down on a bed or the floor, even if you have to crawl there (the only exceptions to this rule are when your leg or legs have suddenly become numb or you have had a fall, accident, or sudden jolt, as described in the questionnaire on the opposite page). Lying down takes the stress off your spine, reducing the pressure to one quarter of that put on it when you are standing. This reduction in pressure may well ease the pain and give the muscles that have gone into a protective spasm the opportunity to relax. You can also help by making a positive mental effort to relax your mind and body and trying not to worry about being inactive – whatever it is that you were doing will have to wait.

THE POSITION TO ADOPT

Lying flat on your back is the most effective way of reducing the pressure on the spine. Try this without a pillow first, but support your head with one if you can still feel the pain; put a pillow under your knees, if necessary, to prevent your lumbar spine from arching too much. If the pain runs down your legs, place a pile of pillows under your lower legs so that your hips and knees are at right angles: this will help relieve pressure on the sciatic nerve (see pages 98-99).

In some cases, lying on your back does not relieve the pain. If you find the position painful, try the maneuvers shown on pages 26-27 to find a position that is pain-free. Answer the questions in the chart on the facing page to find out how serious the problem is likely to be and work out what course of action to take.

HOW SERIOUS IS THE PROBLEM?

Use the questionnaire below to help you decide what to do about your problem – but if you are in any doubt at all, consult your doctor.

1 If any of the following apply, stay absolutely still and ask someone to call an ambulance.

■ You have just been involved in an accident.

■ You have recently had a fall or sudden jolt.

■ One or both of your legs suddenly become numb.

2 If any of the following apply, get medical advice immediately. Telephone your physician or local hospital emergency room.

■ You also have a pain in either your chest, left arm, or jaw.

■ Your pain is unrelenting, growing worse, and not relieved by any change of position.

■ Your legs have felt progressively weaker, with numbness and possible difficulty with urinating and moving your bowels.

■ The pain is continuous, severe, and only relieved by bending forward.

3 If any of the following apply, make an appointment to visit your doctor in the next few days.

■ You also have numbness or pins and needles in the arm or leg.

■ You have lost weight recently and feel generally unwell and tired.

■ You are a woman past menopause.

■ You are pregnant.

■ You are a vegan or you have dieted a lot during your life.

■ You are over 60.

4 If any of the following apply, rest in bed for 24 hours and consult your doctor if there is no improvement after this time.

■ The pain changes if you move or alter position.

■ You have recently done some unaccustomed strenuous exercise.

■ You have twisted suddenly or lifted heavy objects.

2

IMMEDIATE PAIN RELIEF

If you find the position described on page 24 uncomfortable, try the position and exercises below to find a pain-free position in which to rest for 24 hours, but remember that a limited amount of exercise is necessary in order to reduce inflammation and prevent immobilization. As the underlying cause of the pain varies from person to person, you will need to try each position and exercise to find which one helps most in your case – if any part of an exercise maneuver relieves pain, adopt that position for rest. Conversely, don't remain in any position that increases pain. Try the movements in bed if you have a firm mattress; otherwise, use an exercise mat or a thick rug.

A POSITION FOR PAIN RELIEF

1 Lie on your stomach with your hands by your side.

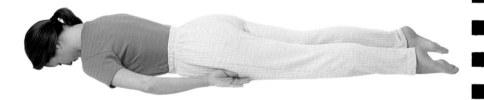

2 If there is still pain, place a pillow under your stomach; if this does not work, try cocking a hip to the side a little – try each hip, because the site of the problem determines which movement is effective. Rest your head on your hands if this is more comfortable.

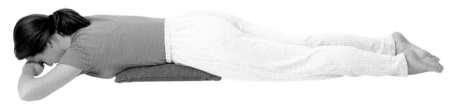

Warning
Stop immediately if any exercise causes or worsens pain or extends its area; otherwise, you may exacerbate the problem. For the first two days, the exercises on these pages should only be repeated three times each, about three times daily, and at other times you should rest. As the pain dies down, gradually increase the number to a maximum of ten repetitions for each exercise.

PELVIC TILTS

1 Lie on your back and bend your knees up at right angles, keeping your feet flat on the floor.

2 Arch the small of your back away from the floor and then push it down hard into the floor. Make sure that your ribcage stays still while your hips rock back and forth.

3 Repeat three times, finishing with the small of the back in a neutral position, halfway between the extremes. Gradually increase the repetitions to ten after the first two days.

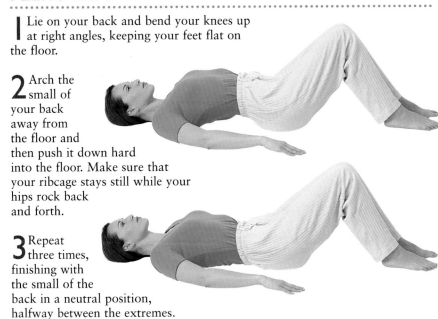

2

KNEE ROLLS

1 Lie on your back and raise your knees, as for the pelvic tilts above, but keep your hips flat on the floor.

2 Rock your knees from side to side, letting them drop as far out toward the ground as is comfortable. Repeat three times, gradually increasing the repetitions to ten after the first two days.

THE SECOND DAY

At one time, doctors thought that complete bed rest was the best treatment for acute back pain, but it has now been shown that a program that mixes exercise and rest is more effective. Call your doctor if there has been no improvement over the first 24 hours, but add the exercises below to those shown on the previous page if the pain has diminished. They will prevent your back from stiffening, which would make chronic problems more likely in the future, and help maintain muscular tone and strength.

PRONE LYING

1 Lie on your stomach on a mat or firm mattress and raise yourself onto your elbows. Relax and hold the position for a count of ten. Relax down, and repeat three times.

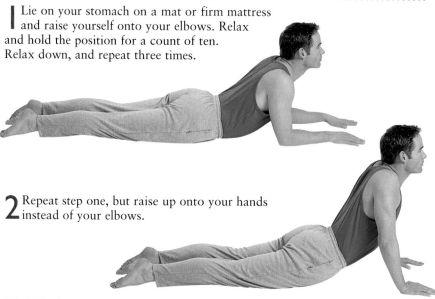

2 Repeat step one, but raise up onto your hands instead of your elbows.

KNEE CURLS

Lie flat on your back on a firm surface, bend your knees to right angles and then pull them up into your chest. Hold for a count of ten and then slowly lower your feet to the ground. Repeat three times.

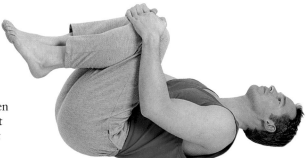

SIDE BENDS

Stand up straight with your feet shoulder width apart. Jut one hip out to the side and slide the arm on the same side down your leg – you will feel a pull on the other side of your body. Repeat three times, then repeat the exercise using the other hip.

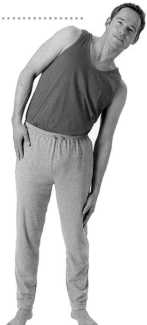

2

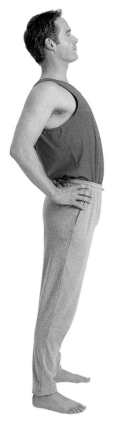

BACK EXTENSION

1 Stand as for the side bends and place your hands on your hips. Arch slightly backward, pulling your shoulder blades together and lifting your chin a little, but not so much that you are looking straight at the ceiling. Repeat three times.

2 After the last repetition, bend slightly forward, curling your shoulders around before finishing in the neutral, upright position.

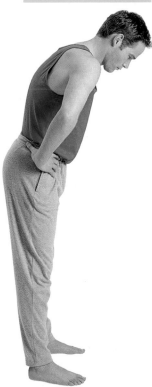

THE ROAD TO RECOVERY

O n the assumption that the pain has continued to diminish – you should consult your doctor if it has not – it is time to resume near-normal life after two days of a mixed program of rest and exercise. It is important that you are as active as possible, in order to restore movement and flexibility, without, of course, doing anything that might impair your recovery. Even so, it is still worthwhile to rest your back for an hour or so each day, to allow the tissues more time to heal and restore themselves.

2

IF THE PAIN RETURNS

Unless you are careful and follow the list of do's and don'ts given on the facing page, there is always a chance that you will make some movement that undoes all the good work and causes your back pain to return. If this happens, stop whatever you are doing and get down onto a firm surface: lie on your face or your back, or adopt whichever position best relieved your pain previously.

LYING ON YOUR SIDE

Lying on your side is not as good for your spine as other positions, but it may be that you are only comfortable if you do so. If this is the case, place a pillow between your knees so your top hip does not roll forward and twist your lower spine. It can also be helpful to place another pillow across the stomach and chest like a bolster – as though you are cuddling it – to support your spine from the front. But avoid having any more than one pillow under your head, especially if the problem is in your neck or upper back.

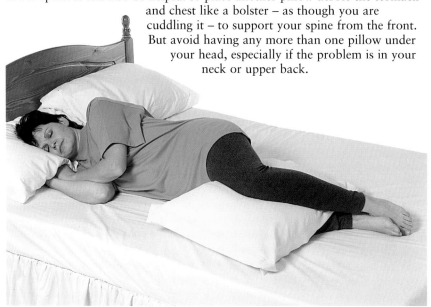

DO'S AND DON'TS FOR RECOVERY

After two days you should get out of bed and do normal everyday things. However, you should bear the following in mind:

Do

■ Continue with your exercises (see pages 26-29) and include exercises to strengthen and improve the flexibility of your spine (see pages 46-55).

■ Check that your posture is correct.

■ Go for walks, extending the distance you walk each day.

■ Resume your normal activities, except those listed under "Don't."

■ Go back to work, unless your job involves lifting and bending.

■ Take frequent breaks if you work at a desk: walk around and arch your back during them (see pages 56-57).

■ Continue making love with your partner, making sure that you use a position that does not cause you pain – perhaps one in which you do not bear any weight. Sexual activity involves movements that are similar to pelvic tilts and can loosen and relax the lower spine.

Don't

■ Don't lift or bend.

■ Don't do heavy housework, such as vacuuming, cleaning, or ironing.

■ Don't walk up or down steep hills.

■ Don't carry heavy objects, such as shopping bags, suitcases, or piles of wet laundry.

■ Don't resume any strenuous sports activities.

■ Don't stand or sit still for long periods of time.

2

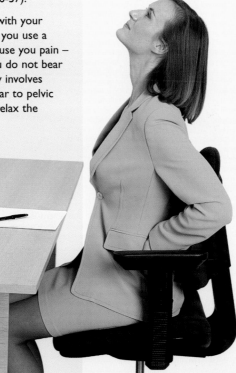

MASSAGE

Massage can be important in the treatment of back problems: it relaxes the muscles of the back and eases any tension, which can either cause back problems or make them worse. A deep massage, though it can sometimes be rather painful, can also break down "trigger points" – particular areas in most large muscles that tend to go into spasm, forming tight knots that hurt if they are touched or rubbed – so that the muscle can regain its smoothness of action and the body can maintain its correct alignment.

2

MASSAGE TECHNIQUE

If you can, visit a professional masseur, who will be experienced in massage skills and techniques. Make sure you tell anyone who is to give you a back massage that you have a back problem and that special care should be taken. You can also have a perfectly good massage at home if you have a willing partner. Make sure the room is warm and lie down on a firm bed or a rug on the floor. Make sure the masseur's hands are warm and covered in massage oil – ordinary baby oil or lotion will do, but add an aromatherapy oil to it for a really relaxing massage. To give a general back massage, ask your partner to do the following:

1 Start at the top of the neck on each side of the spine, then stroke down the center of the back to the buttocks and back up each side, using firm rhythmical strokes. Continue until the whole back has been covered and the recipient is completely relaxed.

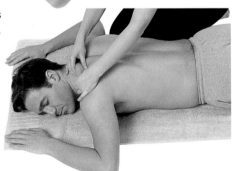

2 Massage the shoulder muscles as though you are kneading dough, paying special attention to any tense or knotted areas. Start near the neck and work out to the tips of the shoulders – generally, it is easier to work on one shoulder at a time. It may be necessary to repeat the massage a few times, since this area holds a lot of tension.

3 Knead the muscles over and around the shoulder blades and the middle of the back, using the same techniques.

4 Start at the neck and circle the thumbs on the band of muscles that run down each side of the spine. Move slowly down the spine, making each stroke overlap on the area covered by the previous one.

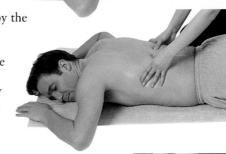

5 Use the whole hand to make large circular movements over the buttocks and back, kneading slightly with the heel of the hand. Finish the massage with long rhythmical strokes over the whole back.

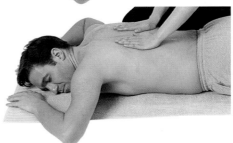

Warning

Do not allow the masseur to press on your spine or manipulate it in any way if any pain runs down your leg or arm.

TRIGGER POINTS

Certain areas in the neck and shoulder muscles tend to go into spasm and become knotted and painful; they are known as "trigger points." Generally, these spasms are caused by habitual poor posture, incorrect use of muscles, or an injury to the neck. Trigger points are very sensitive to touch, and the pain from them tends to radiate out over the neck, head, and shoulders. Although the muscular nodules can be broken down, they will return very quickly unless the root cause of the problem is addressed. The following treatments may be effective:

■ Massage with deep, small, circular movements – known as "friction."

■ The Alexander Technique (see pages 108-109).

■ Injections of anti-inflammatory drugs (see pages 110-111)

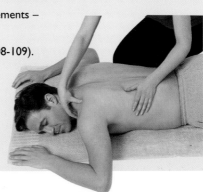

■ Acupuncture (see pages 106-107).

■ Postural correction (see pages 68-71).

■ Physical therapy (see pages 104-105).

AIDS TO SELF-TREATMENT

B ed rest and exercises are not the only form of treatment for acute back pain, though they are essential if recovery is to be complete. Sprays, support devices, and self-massagers can all be used to relieve acute back pain, which is often out of proportion to the damage that has been done to the tissues. The intensity of the pain results from the fact that the muscles that support the spine tend to react to any strain by going into spasm and, in doing so, have a domino effect on other muscles: this gives rise to tension and discomfort in large areas of the back. The aids described here can help to ease muscle tension and relieve pain.

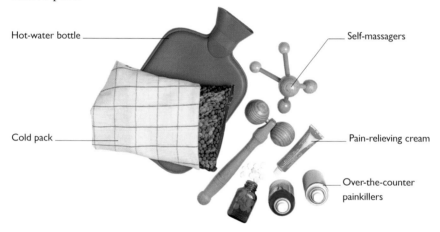

Hot-water bottle

Self-massagers

Cold pack

Pain-relieving cream

Over-the-counter painkillers

HEAT AND COLD

Both heat and cold can ease muscle spasm and tension and so reduce pain. Heat and cold sprays can be bought from most drugstores, but simple measures in the home are just as effective: take a hot bath or apply a hot-water bottle (wrapped in a towel to prevent burns) to the affected area; or use something from the freezer, again, wrapped in a towel – a bag of frozen peas that molds itself to any space is ideal.

SUPPORT SYSTEMS

A doctor or physical therapist may give you a neck collar or a back corset, depending on where the problem is, that gives support to the muscles and joints until the inflammation has died down. Various types of support are available: some inhibit all movement with rigid stays; others are made of flexible foam; and sometimes either type has to be tailor-made to fit the individual concerned. But, unless a doctor or physical therapist recommends otherwise, a support should only be worn as a temporary measure, or the muscles for which it is substituting will weaken as a result of underuse.

MASSAGE MACHINES

Any type of massage helps to relieve muscle tension and, therefore, pain. A professional massage is best (see pages 32-33), but it is also possible to massage yourself using one of the various self-help devices that are available: from wooden beads to battery-operated devices. However, no such devices should be used over the spine itself because of the danger of exacerbating any damage to the vertebrae and disks. Instead, concentrate on any "knots" in the muscles. Battery-operated massagers can also be used to relieve pain by stimulating the skin and overriding pain pathways (see pages 18-20).

CREAMS AND SPRAYS

A number of lotions and sprays can be bought without a doctor's prescription, and all of them claim to ease the pain of muscle tension and muscle spasms. In fact, they do not work on the muscles directly, though they can certainly help relieve pain. Generally, they work by increasing the blood supply to the skin and by "blocking" the pain sensations from the muscles – the sensation of heat is recognized before the sensation of pain by the brain. As the nervous system is unable to recognize these blocked pain impulses, the muscles relax. The muscles stay relaxed until the effect wears off – which is why several applications of cream or spray may be necessary.

OVER-THE-COUNTER MEDICINES

Painkillers, available from any drugstore, are generally very good at doing their job, but in the case of back pain they are just alleviating the effects of the problem rather than making any positive contribution to treating it. The answer is to buy one of the painkillers that contains a muscle relaxant as well as its painkilling ingredient – ask your pharmacist, physical therapist, or doctor for advice on specific brands. This will aid your recovery as well as relieving your pain. But make sure you do not exceed the recommended dose, and always check with your doctor before taking painkillers if you are taking any other medication. Remember, too, that if the painkillers do their job and the pain is relieved, it does not mean that you can return to normal activities immediately: the underlying cause is still present and has merely been disguised.

REGAINING MOBILITY

After about four days of a mixed rest and exercise program, the chances are that you will be free of pain – if not, consult your doctor. So far, the program has been designed to treat acute back pain, but now is the time to start on exercises that will help you regain full mobility. It is vital that you do this, in order to free joints and return muscles and ligaments to their natural state of equilibrium. If the exercises described below are ignored, it is more likely that attacks of acute back pain will recur. Do the exercises described here each morning and evening, but stop immediately if there is any recurrence of the original symptoms. Start your routine with some warm-up exercises (see pages 46-47).

BUTTOCK LIFTS

1 Lie down on your back with your knees at right angles and your feet on the ground.

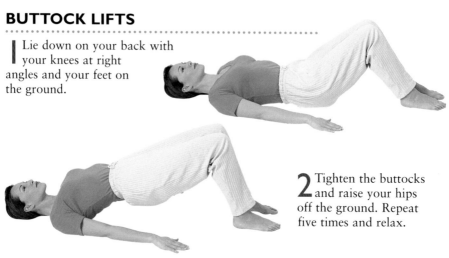

2 Tighten the buttocks and raise your hips off the ground. Repeat five times and relax.

CURL UPS AND KNEE ROLLS

1 Curl your knees into your chest. Repeat five times.

2 Keep your knees curled up on your chest and rock from side to side, with your arms outstretched for balance. Repeat five times and relax.

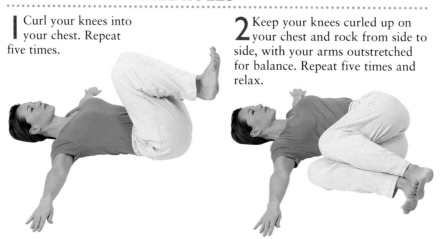

ROCKING

1 Lie on your back with your knees bent, cross your right leg over your left, squeeze your legs together, and tilt them over to the right as far as possible. Repeat five times.

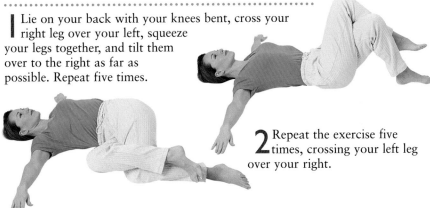

2 Repeat the exercise five times, crossing your left leg over your right.

LEG RAISES

1 Lie on your stomach with your arms by your side.

2 Resting your head on your hands, raise the legs straight up without twisting – expect only a small amount of movement. Repeat five times.

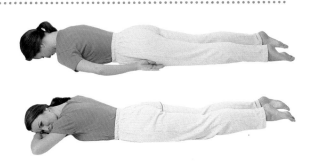

SIDE BEND AND TWIST

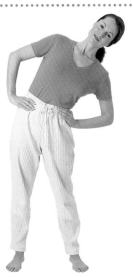

1 Stand with your feet shoulder width apart, place your hands on your hips and tilt over, first to one side and then the other. Do not twist back or forward. Repeat five times for each side, exercising each side alternately.

2 Keeping your hips facing forward, rotate from the waist first to one side and then the other. Repeat five times for each side, exercising each side alternately.

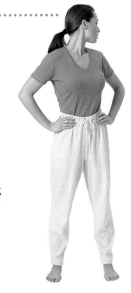

DO'S AND DON'TS

It is important that you strike a balance between regaining mobility and taking care that you do not exacerbate any underlying problem for the first month or so after an attack of acute back pain. Do too much, too quickly, and the problem might recur; do too little and you make it more likely that you will have another attack in the future. Bear in mind the do's and don'ts below.

2

DO'S AND DON'TS FOR REGAINING MOBILITY

Do:

■ Check with your doctor that your back pain has no serious underlying cause.

■ Try to figure out what triggered the attack and modify your lifestyle, if necessary, to avoid it in future.

■ Rest for the first 24 hours following an acute attack of back pain.

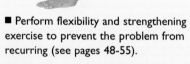
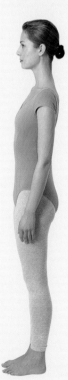

■ Perform flexibility and strengthening exercise to prevent the problem from recurring (see pages 48-55).

■ Make sure you maintain good posture (see pages 68-71).

■ Engage in adequate and frequent exercise.

■ Be careful to follow an exercise correctly when using a home-fitness tape or video.

Don't:

■ Don't embark on an exercise program until you have checked with your doctor that it is safe to do so.

■ Don't perform any high-impact exercises or play high-impact sports, such as tennis, because these place considerable strain on the spine.

■ Don't play sports that involve twisting and bending the spine, such as golf, tennis, racquetball, hockey, football, or baseball.

■ Don't fall into the trap of trying to do too much too soon.

CHRONIC BACK PAIN

Chronic back pain is one of the most common complaints that doctors encounter in industrialized countries. It accounts for more lost working days than any other disorder, and the cost to health-care services is enormous. Yet its causes are often poorly understood. Those who suffer the constant, nagging pain of a bad back, whether continuously or episodically, can find it infuriating that the source of their affliction cannot be identified. But the spine is a complex mechanism, and even minor damage to the joints, muscles, ligaments, and nervous tissues can cause pain. In this chapter, you will find out about the various causes of chronic back pain, what you should do about your pain, and how to condition your body, both to help relieve the pain and to prevent it from recurring.

3

MUSCULAR CAUSES

The most common cause of chronic back pain is that the vertebral column, or a part of it, has been compressed too much, with the result that each vertebra is squashed down onto the next one. This causes the intervertebral disks to lose their sponginess and shrink; the bones of the facet joints become jammed too close together; and the edges of the vertebrae either wear away or grow small, bony spurs called osteophytes (see page 95). Muscular problems are a common reason for compression and may themselves result from a lack of exercise, poor posture, an imbalance in the muscles, and abdominal weakness: these problems are described here.

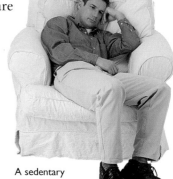

LACK OF EXERCISE

If muscles are not used regularly, they lose their ability to contract fully and become weak. This means that they can no longer maintain enough tension to play their part in the complex network of tissues that support the spine and maintain it in its correct position. Regular light exercise is enough to keep the muscles in good working order (see pages 46-59).

A sedentary lifestyle makes chronic back pain much more likely.

3

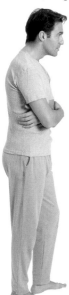

POOR POSTURE

Any posture that changes the spine's natural curves causes muscular changes that tend to make the variation permanent (see pages 68-71). A change to the spine's natural curves compresses the intervertebral disks so they start to shrink and lose their elasticity. The muscles change because they work in pairs: as one muscle group contracts, another group, opposing it, relaxes. For example, if you spend too much time stooping over, the pectoral muscles – on the chest – will stay contracted, while the muscles of the upper back relax. Over time, the pectorals will become stronger and the upper back muscles weaker, pulling the spine out of alignment. Your back will become rounded, the pressure on the spine will be uneven, and a chronic back problem will be the result.

MUSCULAR IMBALANCE

Unless you are ambidextrous, you will not use each arm to the same degree. As a result, the muscles on one side of the body become more developed than the other. In some cases – for example, with avid tennis or racquetball players – the extra strength of the overdeveloped side of the body can pull the spine out of alignment so that when viewed from the back it is not straight but has a "C" or an "S" bend (see page 100). This is an extreme example, but even a minor difference in the strength of different sides of the body will affect the thoracic spine.

The spine may appear to be straight, but the pressure on the vertebrae and intervertebral disks will be unequal. Over time, the disk will be squashed on the stronger side; the vertebra will suffer from more wear and tear on that side; and the facet joint may become jammed.

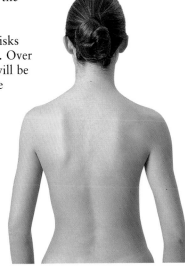

ABDOMINAL WEAKNESS

Strong abdominal muscles act as a corset and hold the abdominal contents close to the spine. Normally this corset bears some of the body's weight, relieving the pressure on the spine and hips. However, any weakness in the abdominal muscles, which may be the result of lack of exercise or of being overweight or pregnant, puts the pressure back onto the lumbar spine. The result can be an excessive forward curve in the region, called a lordosis (see page 101), that will eventually cause chronic back pain.

BACK PAIN AND DISEASE

Chronic back pain is sometimes a symptom or a consequence of some other disease. For this reason it is important to consult a doctor in all cases of chronic back pain, in order to rule out the presence of an underlying disorder. Medical conditions that can cause chronic back pain include:

- Ankylosing spondylitis (see page 101).

- Cancer.

- Gynecological problems (low back pain).

- Kidney infections (low back pain).

- Osteomalacia.

- Osteoporosis (see page 96).

- Rheumatoid arthritis.

- Spondylolisthesis.

- Stomach and gallbladder problems (thoracic spine pain).

3

SKELETAL CAUSES

When skeletal problems are the root cause of chronic back pain, the responsibility for damage to the bones and joints generally lies with the degenerative processes involved in aging – though on rare occasions an underlying medical disorder may be to blame. "Wear and tear" is not always the culprit, however: sometimes unnatural strains on the spine can also damage joints and so contribute to the problem.

DISK SHRINKAGE

The intervertebral disks, which are largely composed of water, play a vital role in enabling the spine to turn, twist, and arch (see page 13). However, with age – as part of the natural process of osteoarthritis – the water content of the disks diminishes; this process can, however, be slowed down (see page 94). The result is that the disks gradually lose their bounce and spring so that by old age they are often much thinner and weaker than before. Certain factors accelerate the loss: inadequate movement of the spine; prolonged, uneven pressure on the disk; continual pressure, for example, as a result of sitting still for long periods; and inadequate rest.

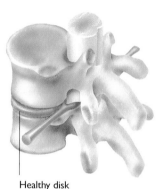

Healthy disk

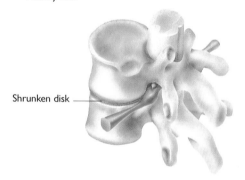

Shrunken disk

HOW DAMAGED DISKS CAUSE PAIN

As the disks lose their high water content, the fibrous ring that encircles them becomes more brittle and often develops cracks through which the inner gelatinous fluid oozes. Sometimes this does not itself cause any pain, but, depending on the site of the leak, the fluid may press against a ligament, the dura (the layers that surround the spinal cord), or a spinal nerve. If this is the case, there may be a chronic ache at the site of the problem or severe "referred" pain elsewhere in the body – that is, pain in an area supplied by the spinal nerve that is being compressed by the fluid. Even if the inner fluid does not escape, the fibrous ring may be weakened to such an extent that the walls of the disk bulge out under the continuous downward pressure of the body's weight, causing similar problems.

FACET JOINT PROBLEMS

Chronic back pain is often caused by damage to the facet joints, on the upper and lower surfaces of the vertebrae that link each vertebra to the next one in the column. The surfaces of these joints are covered with cartilage, which reduces friction, and lubricated with synovial fluid, which is contained within a fibrous capsule surrounding the joint. In order to work efficiently, the two opposing bones have to glide smoothly over each other. However, if they are pressed together too tightly, as happens when the spine is compressed, the cartilaginous linings become worn, and the joint becomes inflamed as a result.

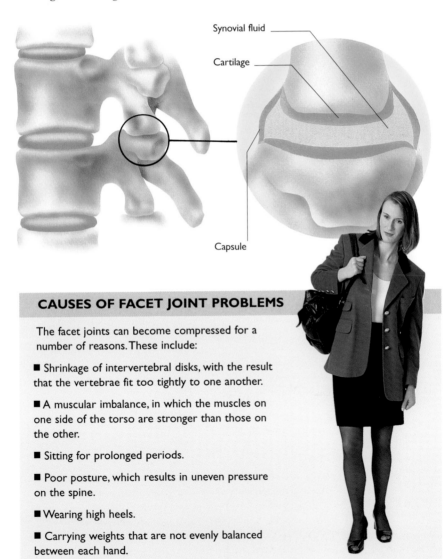

Synovial fluid

Cartilage

Capsule

3

CAUSES OF FACET JOINT PROBLEMS

The facet joints can become compressed for a number of reasons. These include:

■ Shrinkage of intervertebral disks, with the result that the vertebrae fit too tightly to one another.

■ A muscular imbalance, in which the muscles on one side of the torso are stronger than those on the other.

■ Sitting for prolonged periods.

■ Poor posture, which results in uneven pressure on the spine.

■ Wearing high heels.

■ Carrying weights that are not evenly balanced between each hand.

WHAT TO DO ABOUT IT

It cannot be emphasized too strongly that anyone who suffers from chronic back pain should consult a doctor to rule out the possibility of an underlying medical disorder. That having been said, there is much that you can do to relieve chronic back pain that arises from muscular or skeletal problems. Unless an underlying disorder is involved, you should adopt the program of exercises for increasing the flexibility and strength of your back that is given on the following pages. However, before undertaking the program, you should ask your doctor for confirmation that it is suitable in your particular case.

3

DEALING WITH CHRONIC BACK PAIN

Chronic pain of any kind can be profoundly depressing. However, it is important to try to develop a positive attitude to overcoming your back problem. You may not feel the benefit immediately, but in time the exercises given in the following pages – which should always be preceded by a warm-up (see pages 46-47) – will help to restore flexibility and strength to your spine if performed every day, and so help prevent the recurrence of any problem. However, exercise alone is not always enough to relieve pain completely. This is because other factors, apart from purely mechanical and physical ones, are at work in many cases.

If you suffer from chronic back pain, you may find that using a cane makes walking more comfortable. Be sure to use it correctly. Seek advice from your doctor or physical therapist.

Warning

If you feel an increase in any pain while doing the exercises on the pages that follow, or if it returns, stop what you are doing immediately. Rest in a pain-free position and review the situation: you might have overdone things and caused an attack of acute back pain (see page 24).

WHY CHRONIC BACK PAIN TENDS TO LINGER

Chronic back pain has a notorious tendency to linger with debilitating effects for months and even years. There are three main reasons for this:

Reason for pain	How problem is caused	How to overcome the problem
Overuse of prescribed or over-the-counter painkillers.	Some painkillers work by reproducing the effects of endorphins, the body's own painkilling chemicals (see page 20). During their use, the normal production of endorphins is reduced; and when painkillers are stopped, the body takes time to produce natural endorphins in adequate quantities again.	Use painkillers only during an acute attack of back pain, unless you have been advised to take them for longer by your doctor. Instead, try to rely on a mixture of rest in a pain-free position and gentle exercises to alleviate pain. Use deep relaxation to boost the release of natural endorphins.
A heightened perception of pain or a low pain threshold.	Stress and depression caused by the pain of a chronic back problem and by its effects, such as inactivity and a restricted social life, often tend to make people feel pain more keenly. This in turn reinforces the depressive effect, because every twinge is a reminder that the problem has still not gone away.	Take positive steps to relax and get enough rest and sleep (see page 84). At the same time, try to resume normal activities as soon as you can, in order to combat stress and depression. In the short term, you may need to adapt your activities according to the restrictions created by your back problem.
Pain gates (see pages 18-20) are open all the time.	This can occur as a result of the gateways being bombarded by signals. This means that more pain impulses can pass through unblocked, and more pain is felt.	The healing effects of exercise and massage can help to restore the normal functioning of the pain gateways.

3

WARM-UP EXERCISES

A warm-up routine boosts the supply of blood and oxygen to the muscles, tendons, and ligaments. This makes them more supple and flexible and so more efficient and less prone to strains; it also increases the speed of nerve transmissions to the muscles. As a result, a good warm-up is in itself an important part of a back-care regime. However, it is vital that you warm up properly before undertaking the flexibility and strengthening exercises on the following pages, in order to minimize the risk of damaging the tissues even more. Use it, too, once the chronic pain has passed, before you engage in strenuous activities around the home, such as gardening or heavy housework, in order to help prevent a recurrence of the problem.

STRETCHING AND LOOSENING

Stand straight, with your feet the width of your shoulders apart. Then go through the following exercises, repeating each one five times.

1 Start the warm-up by taking two deep breaths and exhaling them, emptying the lungs completely.

2 Shrug your shoulders up and down and then circle backward and forward.

3 Turn your head from side to side; then up and down.

4 Swing your arms up and back in ever-increasing circles.

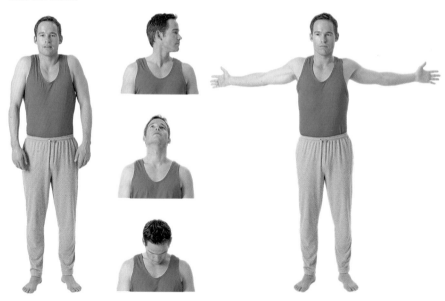

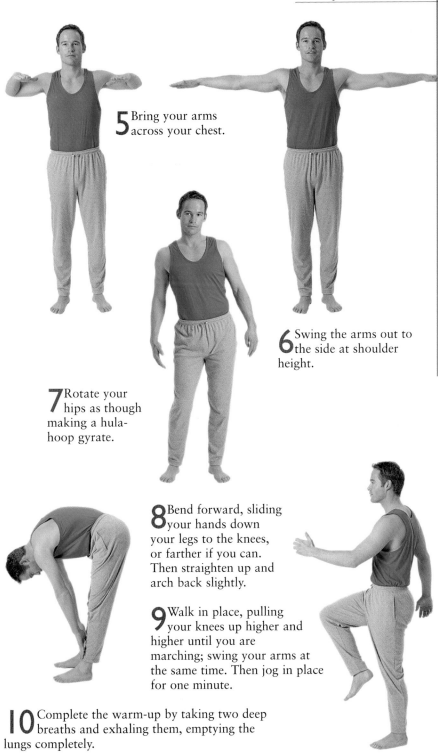

5 Bring your arms across your chest.

6 Swing the arms out to the side at shoulder height.

3

7 Rotate your hips as though making a hula-hoop gyrate.

8 Bend forward, sliding your hands down your legs to the knees, or farther if you can. Then straighten up and arch back slightly.

9 Walk in place, pulling your knees up higher and higher until you are marching; swing your arms at the same time. Then jog in place for one minute.

10 Complete the warm-up by taking two deep breaths and exhaling them, emptying the lungs completely.

FLEXIBILITY EXERCISES: 1

A supple back can absorb the stresses and strains of everyday movements. These exercises increase suppleness and flexibility by keeping the intervertebral joints and facet joints well lubricated and moving freely. Flexing both the large and small back muscles makes them less likely to go into spasm, which is one of the prime causes of chronic back pain.

FLEXING MUSCLES AND LUBRICATING JOINTS

Kneel on a carpet or a mat and perform these exercises, repeating each one five times. It is best to go through the whole routine every morning and every evening, and make it part of your life, even when the chronic pain has gone.

3

I Get down on all fours with your hips and shoulders at right angles to each other.

REMEMBER TO WARM UP AND COOL DOWN

It is vital that you do a warm-up routine (see pages 46-47) before undertaking any of these exercises – and it is also useful to do one before setting about any heavy work around the home, such as gardening or cleaning. Cool down when you have finished the exercises by repeating the warm-up exercises.

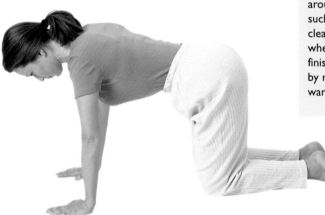

2 Drop your head down to your knees, keeping your hands and knees still and rounding your back, then uncurl.

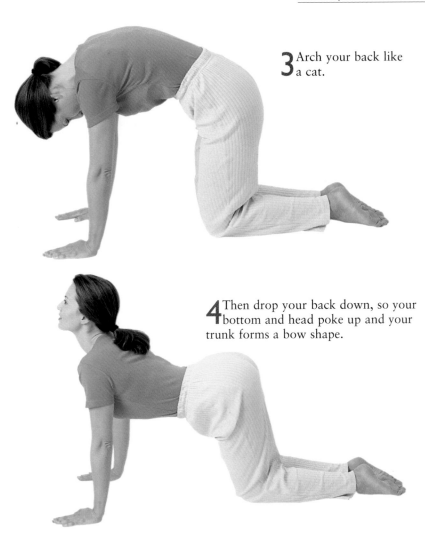

3 Arch your back like a cat.

4 Then drop your back down, so your bottom and head poke up and your trunk forms a bow shape.

3

5 Keeping your back straight, raise the opposite arm and leg straight out in front of you and behind you, respectively. Repeat with the other arm and leg.

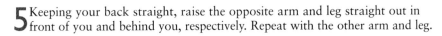

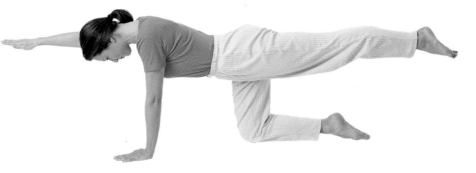

FLEXIBILITY EXERCISES: 2

The exercises on these pages not only improve the flexibility of your spine but, since they are carried out when standing, help improve your general posture by easing any stiffness or tension in the muscles. In addition, they increase the range of movement in the spinal joints, making an injury less likely when bending, stretching, or lifting.

INCREASING FLEXIBILITY AND THE RANGE OF MOVEMENT

Repeat the exercises below five times each morning and evening, even after the pain has gone. Start by standing on the floor or a mat with your feet the width of your shoulders apart and your elbows bent up at right angles.

3

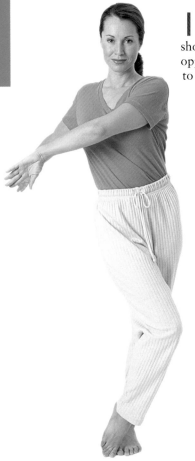

1 Swing your arms and shoulders in the opposite direction to your hips.

2 Pull your shoulders and arms back so the palms of your hands face out to the side.

3 Then stick your bottom out and round your shoulders – your hands will now turn in and back. Then curl your bottom under.

4 Kneel down, sitting on your ankles. Using your arms for balance, move your bottom over to the right so your right hip is resting on the floor and your arms are to your left. Then raise your bottom and sit on the other side, changing the arms to the right. Repeat six times, moving three times in each direction.

3

REMEMBER TO WARM UP AND COOL DOWN

It is vital that you do a warm-up routine (see pages 46-47) before undertaking any of these exercises – and it is also useful to do one before setting about any heavy work around the home, such as gardening or cleaning. Cool down when you have finished the exercises by repeating the warm-up exercises.

5 Stand up and move to a horizontal pole or a door frame. Grasp it with your hands and let it take all the weight of your body. Let your knees give way so you can feel your spine stretching. Hold for 30 seconds and relax. Let go of the pole and stand normally.

BACK STRENGTHENING: 1

The muscles of the stomach and back must not only be flexible but also strong, if they are to give the spine adequate support. Weak muscles cannot bear their proper share of the stresses and strains that the back must withstand, which means that joints and ligaments of the spine have to do more than their fair share of the work. These do not have as good a blood supply as the muscles, and, over time, wear and tear in them is accelerated, leading to tissue damage and chronic back pain. However, exercises that strengthen the muscles can help relieve pain by giving them the ability to take on more of the stresses and strains and so reduce the demands on the joints and ligaments.

STEPS TO BUILDING UP BACK STRENGTH

Lie on a carpet or a mat – you will need a table for the Leg Raises – and perform the exercises below, repeating each one five times. Make them part of your morning and evening routine, and keep going after the pain has gone – doing so will help prevent any recurrence of the problem.

3

BACK ARCHES

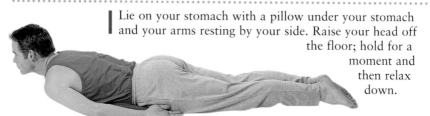

1 Lie on your stomach with a pillow under your stomach and your arms resting by your side. Raise your head off the floor; hold for a moment and then relax down.

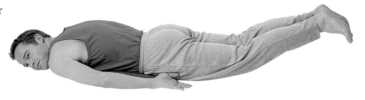

2 Relax your shoulders and raise your legs 6 inches off the ground.

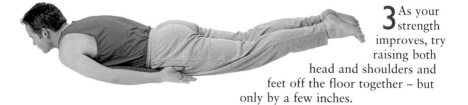

3 As your strength improves, try raising both head and shoulders and feet off the floor together – but only by a few inches.

BACK CURLS

1 Lie on your back and curl up, reaching with your hands for your knees.

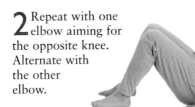

2 Repeat with one elbow aiming for the opposite knee. Alternate with the other elbow.

3 As your strength improves, raise the opposite knee to meet the elbow. Exercise alternate sides.

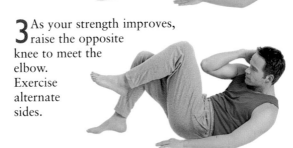

3

LEG RAISES

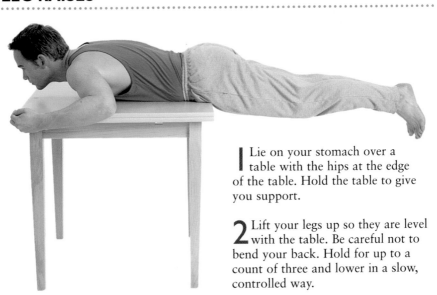

1 Lie on your stomach over a table with the hips at the edge of the table. Hold the table to give you support.

2 Lift your legs up so they are level with the table. Be careful not to bend your back. Hold for up to a count of three and lower in a slow, controlled way.

BACK STRENGTHENING: 2

As your back and stomach muscles gain in strength, you will find that daily tasks are easier to perform and that your general posture is well on the way to improving to such an extent that a chronic back problem is much less likely to recur. Now is the time to move on to the more demanding exercises shown on these pages, in order to consolidate your improvement. Do not attempt these exercises unless you have spent some time doing the ones on the previous pages and can complete them with ease – this may take a few weeks. As before, repeat each exercise five times, morning and night, and continue with this routine even after any pain has gone.

LEG LIFTS

1 Lie on your side, with the lower arm under your head and the other resting in front of you to give stability. Bend your lower leg and raise your upper leg straight up, with the foot flexed rather than pointed.

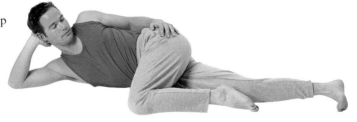

2 Drop the top leg forward onto the floor. Rest your arm on your hip.

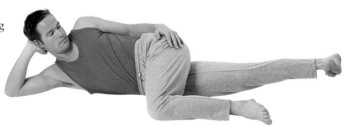

3 Raise the underneath leg a little way off the ground. Turn over, and repeat the above exercises when lying on the other side.

SIT-UPS

1 Sit on the floor with your knees bent at right angles to your chest. Hold your arms out in front for balance.

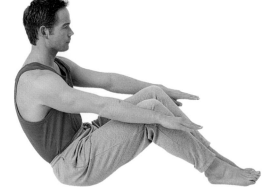

2 Controlling the movement with your stomach muscles, rock back as far as comfortable.

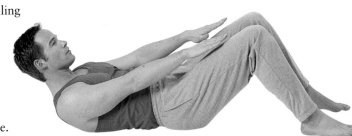

3 Continuing to use your stomach muscles, pull right up.

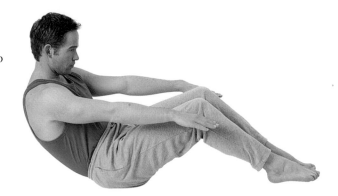

3

REMEMBER TO WARM UP AND COOL DOWN

It is vital that you do a warm-up routine (see pages 46-47) before undertaking any of these exercises – and it is also useful to do one before setting about any heavy work around the home, such as gardening or cleaning. Cool down when you have finished the exercises by repeating the warm-up exercises.

STRETCHES

One of the problems of modern life is that, for the majority of people, most of the day is spent in a sedentary position – whether sitting at a desk, using a computer, or driving. This tends to make the back stiffen up, especially if it is already prone to problems, and this can undo all the good work that has been put in previously. The stretches shown below can be used to prevent your back from stiffening up.

STRETCHES FOR REGULAR AND EMERGENCY USE

These stretches only take a few minutes, and it is well worth doing some of them on a regular basis – after every hour spent sitting, say. They can also be used in an emergency, when your back is beginning to stiffen up and is starting to ache. Repeat each stretch five times, and choose the ones that are easiest to do, in practical terms, given your work environment. As an alternative to the pelvic tilts in a sitting position, you could try them in a lying-down position, as described on page 27.

BACK FLEXIONS

1 Lie on your side and curl up as tightly as possible into a ball. Feel the pull on your spine.

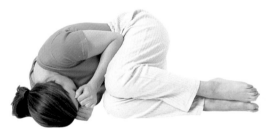

Warning

If any of these movements aggravates any ache or pain or widens its area, stop immediately and rest in the position that you have previously found to be pain-free.

2 Stretch back out slowly and gently, extending your arms above your head, straightening your legs and pointing your toes.

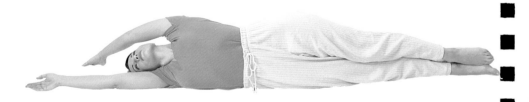

PELVIC TILTS: SITTING

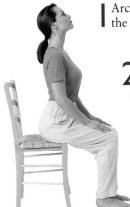

1 Arch your back away from the back of the chair.

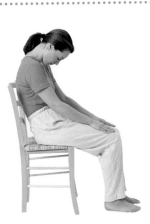

2 Then roll it back so it presses against the chair once more. After five repetitions, finish with the small of your back in a neutral position, halfway between the two extremes.

PELVIC TILTS: STANDING

1 Put your hands on your hips and arch your back, tilting your pelvis forward.

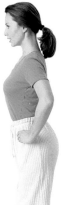

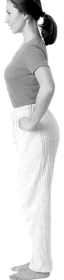

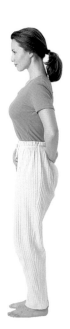

2 Then tilt your pelvis back and tuck your bottom in. Finish with your back in a neutral position, halfway between the two extremes.

KNEE ROLLS

1 Lie on your back with your knees bent up to your chest and arms stretched out to the sides.

3

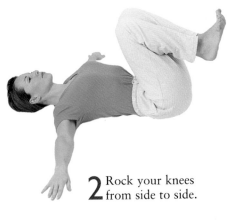

2 Rock your knees from side to side.

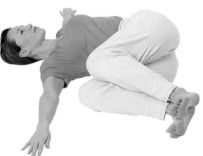

GENERAL FITNESS

There is only one way to achieve general physical fitness, and that is by exercising regularly. And it is well worth doing so, because being fit is not only good for general health, and reducing the risk of a number of diseases and problems at any age, but has a direct effect on the well-being of your back. Some people find that the discipline of joining a gym or a fitness class helps them become fit, but it is not necessary to do so. The most important thing is to do some form of exercise at least three times a week – whether it be a vigorous walk, a bicycle ride, or a few lengths of the swimming pool. However, don't play sports that put strain on the back, such as racquetball and tennis, or try high-impact aerobics until you have achieved a good level of overall fitness.

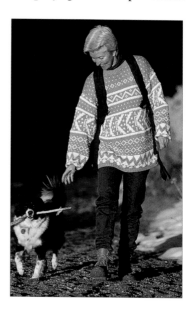

MENTAL BENEFITS

Many people think of exercise and general fitness as something that is only important for the body. But, in fact, it has a pervasive benefit on both mind and body. Exercise can reduce stress levels, both in terms of mental stress and its physical manifestations. For example, mental stress often affects the trapezius, a muscle at the back of the neck: certain fibers in the muscle knot under stress, and these areas, known as "trigger points," can prevent the muscle from relaxing (see page 33).

Warning

Fitness should be built up gradually and over time. Inappropriate and excessive exercise can cause damage, including:

- Muscle, tendon, and ligament strains and tears.

- Stress on the joints.

- Inflammation of tendons and joint capsules.

- Aches, pains, and stiffness.

Do not embark on a strenuous exercise program, especially if you have previously been living a sedentary life, without first consulting your doctor.

PHYSICAL BENEFITS

Regular exercise, resulting in good physical fitness, has a number of beneficial effects on the body and its organs. These include:

■ A stronger heart and a lower pulse rate. Exercise increases the size of the heart so it can pump out more blood with each beat. This means that it has to beat less often, with the result that the pulse rate decreases – an average pulse rate is around 74 beats per minute, but highly trained athletes have pulse rates as low as 45 beats per minute.

■ Improved breathing and lung function. Exercise increases the volume of air breathed in, which increases both the elasticity of lung tissue and the blood supply to the lungs. Deeper breathing also increases the stamina and strength of the muscles that move the ribcage and support the thoracic spine.

■ Improved muscle tone, strength, and stamina, which in turn promote good posture and body shape. Both muscle strengthening and flexibility exercises (see pages 48-55) increase the amount of energy stored in the muscles, with the result that they can react quickly to any demands and are less likely to be damaged by any sudden movement or wrench. Strong, flexible muscles also provide good support for the spine.

■ Tendons and ligaments that increase their tensile strength and become more resilient to strain. This increases the range of movement at joints and reduces the likelihood of tissue damage.

■ The increased production of synovial fluid in certain joints, such as the facet joints of the spine. This nourishes and lubricates the articulating cartilage, so wear and tear is reduced.

■ Strong bones, developed and maintained by weight-bearing exercise. This helps combat osteoporosis (see page 96) and is a vital form of exercise for post-menopausal women, in particular.

■ Reduced reaction time, improved balance and coordination.

3

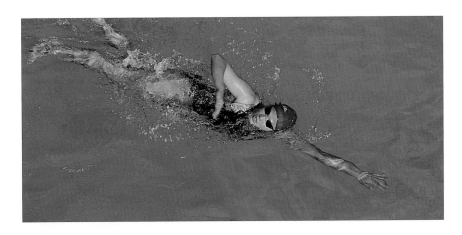

AVOIDING STRAIN

Most people never pay a thought to their backs until they have had an attack of acute back pain or have become aware of the onset of chronic pain. For this reason, a certain amount of damage has normally been done by the time a problem is recognized. Much of this damage is reversible, but there is often some residual weakness. This makes it important for anyone who has had a back problem to take steps to reduce the chance of any recurrence by paying due care and attention to avoiding back strain.

AVOIDING STRAIN WHEN DRIVING

Driving long distances gives most people backache whether they have a back problem or not. Driving entails small movements in a flexed position, which automatically puts the spine under stress – and until recently, most car seats were not designed to help.

■ Adjust the car seat and angle of the back rest until the steering wheel and gear lever and pedals can be reached comfortably with the knees slightly bent and the thighs level. If the seat has no lumbar support, place a small pillow at your lower back. The seat should be firm and supportive. The back rest should be high and wide enough to support the upper body and prevent you from being thrown sideways when turning corners.

■ Car accessory stores sell many aids for comfort, such as lumbar supports and wooden bead covers, but if these do not help and you suffer from a chronic back problem, it may be worth changing your car to a model that gives more support and comfort. It is no use sitting in a car in a showroom since it is not only the flexed position but the driving itself that produces the problem. Ask whether you can test drive the car for at least half an hour.

■ Getting in and out of a car can be difficult. Try to avoid any twisting. Move the car seat as far back as possible and swing your legs and body around in one movement before standing up to get out. Use the reverse movement to get in.

HIGH HEELS

Avoid high heels whenever possible, because they cause the curve at the base of the spine to increase. This not only compresses the vertebrae but stretches the abdominal muscles and throws the contents of the abdomen forward. The effect is to reduce the intra-abdominal pressure with the result that the spine has less support at the front of the body.

TEN STEPS TO BACK PROTECTION

It may seem difficult to keep all these measures in mind throughout a busy working day, but if you persevere, they will become a habit and considerably reduce the chances that your back problem will recur.

1 Check your posture at frequent intervals through the day, especially when at work, so that correct posture becomes a habit.

2 Avoid holding any position that causes tension in your back muscles – as, for example, when bending over a workbench or washing your hair in a sink. Bad posture when you are in a static position causes muscles to become tense and ache and ligaments to become stretched and painful. This is likely, in turn, to make muscle fibers go into spasm and for some of them to form tight, painful, knotted joints.

3 Avoid standing still for any length of time. If this proves impossible, do some stretches (see pages 56-57) or rest one leg on a stool or bar to ease the strain on your lower back.

4 Warm up (see pages 46-47) before doing any exercise or before any heavy work around the home, such as gardening.

5 Exercise to keep your back and abdominal muscles strong and flexible (see pages 48-55), since the spine becomes unstable and is injured easily if its muscular support is inadequate.

6 Make sure you weigh the correct amount for your height, build, and age, and maintain this weight (see pages 80-83).

7 Make sure you have ample sleep and rest, since the intervertebral disks reabsorb the water they lose in the course of daily activities during these times.

8 Avoid making two movements at the same time, especially if different muscle groups are being used. For example, do not lift a heavy weight while twisting your body – as happens when taking a child out of a car seat.

9 Take time to relax during the day in order to release the muscle tensions that build up, especially around the neck.

10 If you have to carry heavy loads, make sure the weight is evenly distributed between the two sides of your body (see page 76). Asymmetrical loads cause the stress to be unevenly distributed down the spine, with the result that one side is under more pressure than the other.

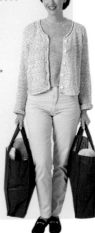

3

ADAPTING YOUR HOME

Long-term sufferers from chronic back pain may have to accept that some permanent damage has been done to the spine and that they are likely to suffer from bouts of discomfort and pain. If this is the case, you should adapt your environment in order to reduce the amount of stress that is put on your back – the kitchen being the main area of concern. You will still be able to live an active life, and you will suffer from attacks of pain less frequently.

ADAPTING YOUR KITCHEN

Most people spend a surprising amount of time in the kitchen, and unfortunately, it is full of hazards for back sufferers. For example, work surfaces tend to be a standard height from the ground, and usually they are far too low. Lifting heavy cooking utensils, too, can cause back strains – especially when they are stored in high or low cupboards.

WORK SURFACES

Check the height of your work surfaces. Ideally, the top of the surface should be 3 inches lower than your elbow so you can prepare food without stooping. In the majority of kitchens, the surfaces are likely to need to be raised by at least 6 inches for use by a woman and by more to be correct for a man. Installing new surfaces is an expensive option, but you can make at least one area the correct height: buy a large, oblong chopping board and raise it on blocks to the correct height; or raise one or two of your units by putting them on a plinth – remember not to do this yourself.

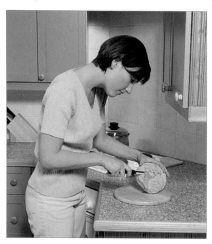

When the work surface is too low, you are forced to work with a bent back.

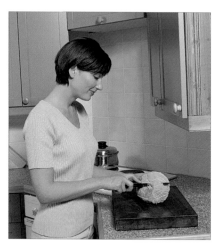

A raised work surface means you can keep your back straight and relaxed.

WASHING DISHES

When you are washing dishes, you can avoid back strain by raising the level at which you are working. Place a plastic tub upside down in the sink and stand another one on top of it; this should allow you to work at a more suitable height. Stand as close to the sink as you can. Opening the cabinet door under the sink may allow you to get closer.

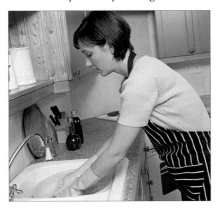

When the sink is too low, you have to lean over, causing back strain.

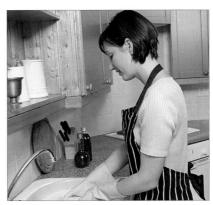

Standing close to a raised washing tub allows your back to remain upright.

3

STORAGE

■ Put things that you use frequently within easy reach on the work surface. Ask someone else to pull heavy dishes out from high cupboards the evening or morning before you need them and remember to kneel to get utensils from a floor cupboard.

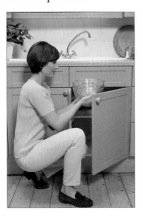

■ Heavy kitchen equipment, such as a food processor, should be left in one position and not put away.

■ Even filling a jug can cause problems when your back is weak: instead, fill a small pitcher with water and transfer the water to the jug by pitcher.

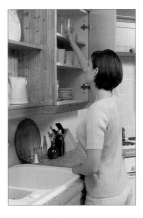

Bend your knees, rather than your back, to pick up heavy items from floor cupboards.

Keep only light items on high shelves. Heavy items should be kept within easy reach.

HOUSEWORK TECHNIQUES

Never try to do all the housework in one day if you suffer from back problems. Instead, work out a system by which you do a little each day. Stop frequently to take a break, and never struggle on until the pain forces you to stop. If possible, persuade your partner or a friend to take care of heavy jobs, such as putting out the trash and carrying shopping bags. If this is not possible, take heavy jobs very slowly, bit by bit – even if they take longer to complete.

GENERAL HOUSEWORK

For safety, do a warm-up routine (see pages 46-47) before you start any housework. The most important thing to remember is to take everything slowly and to vary the muscle groups that you are using – do not continue with just one activity or the same type of pressure will be on the spine for too long. For example, it is better to clean one room at a time, so that you do some vacuuming, some polishing, and some dusting, rather than, for example, vacuuming the whole house in one day. And when you polish or dust, try to use alternate hands so the strain is symmetrical and balanced. If you find this impossible, even after practice, pretend to polish or dust with your other hand so at least the same muscles are exercised on each side of the body.

IRONING

Ironing can place considerable strain on the spine, because your arms are exerting a downward pressure in front of you as you stoop over the board. To keep the stress to a minimum:

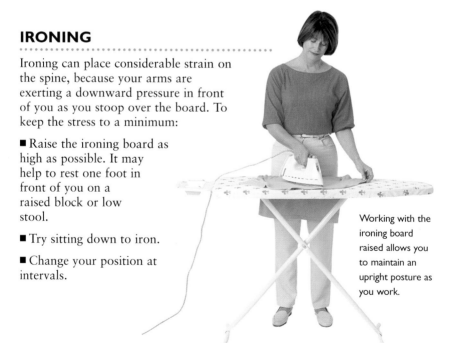

■ Raise the ironing board as high as possible. It may help to rest one foot in front of you on a raised block or low stool.

■ Try sitting down to iron.

■ Change your position at intervals.

Working with the ironing board raised allows you to maintain an upright posture as you work.

DOING THE LAUNDRY

It is easy to forget that a pile of wet laundry can be fairly heavy, so bear in mind the following:

■ Remember to kneel down to put clothes in and take clothes out of a washing machine or dryer.

■ Only put a few clothes in a laundry basket at a time – make return trips to and from the machine if necessary.

■ Take only a few items at a time to hang up on a clothes line, and make sure the line is at a sensible height so you do not have to stretch up.

VACUUMING

Cleaning the carpets is a routine chore but one that can demand a fair amount of strength, even in the cleanest house. Unfortunately, it may also demand a stooping position, which can injure the back. Remember the following:

■ Use an upright model of vacuum cleaner.

■ Keep the vacuum cleaner close to your body and use small sweeps, so you do not have to bend.

■ Alternate the use of your hands.

■ Take frequent breaks.

3

MAKING THE BED

Most people prefer to get into a neat, well-made bed when they are ready to go to sleep. Unfortunately, though, making a bed involves a considerable amount of stooping and lifting. If you do not have anyone to help you make the bed, follow these guidelines to avoid exacerbating a back problem:

■ Buy a bed that is high off the ground (see page 86) – a high bed requires less bending to make.

■ Ideally, buy fitted sheets and a comforter.

■ Bend your knees or kneel on the floor to tuck sheets in.

■ Never stretch over a bed to tuck in the other side. Instead, position the bed so you have all-round access.

■ Make sure other members of the household make and change the sheets on their own beds.

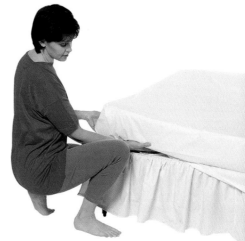

BATHROOM TIPS

It is easy to forget to think about protecting your back in the morning as you rush to get on with the day – even if you may feel that it has stiffened overnight, as often happens with age. The trouble is that a bad start to the day, in which you put extra stresses on the spine, can lead to hours of back pain – and stooping over when your hands are raised, to shave, wash you hair, or put on make-up, makes this only too likely. Try to give yourself enough time in the morning so you do not have to rush and can take proper precautions.

BACK SAFETY WATCHPOINTS

The key to avoiding straining your back in the bathroom is to remember not to stoop if you can avoid it. Bear these points in mind:

■ Have a shower instead of a bath, if possible – you will not have to stoop when taking a shower.

■ Make sure the shaving or make-up mirror is accessible enough that you do not have to bend forward to see it properly – buy an extending mirror if necessary.

■ Do not wash your hair in a sink since you will have to stoop over too much while your hands are raised. Instead, wash your hair in the shower or kneel at the edge of the bathtub. In the latter case, use a hand-held shower attachment to rinse your hair.

■ A warm bath can be very relaxing for the back muscles, but try to avoid having the lumbar spine too rounded. A bath head pillow may help with upper back and neck pain.

■ Be careful when you get out of the bathtub: stand up first and then step out; otherwise, you will be straining up and twisting at the same time. Handrails halfway down the bathtub can help you do this, and a bath mat will prevent you from slipping.

■ Sit down to dry your feet and pull each foot up rather than bending over to it. If you find this impossible, you may find it easier to stand on a towel and work it over the top of both feet.

■ Leaning over to clean the tub can easily strain a vulnerable back, so try to persuade someone else to clean it for you if you can. Otherwise, kneel on the floor as close to the edge of the tub as possible, use a spray or foam cleanser, and rinse it off with a hand-held shower attachment.

■ Avoid using oils in the bathtub since they make the bath more slippery, increasing the risk of injury through falls. Oils also tend to make the tub more troublesome to clean.

PREVENTING BACK PROBLEMS

Whether or not you are currently suffering from back problems, you can avoid exacerbating chronic aches and pains and reduce the risk of suffering an acute back problem by taking a few simple preventive measures. Pay close attention to your posture, both when sitting and standing, and take practical measures to make sure your working environment does not put any unnecessary strain on your back, and approach any task that might strain your back – such as lifting a heavy object or gardening – in the correct manner. This section of the book tells you why you should adopt these measures and how to do so. It also looks at how your weight, your ability to relax, and your sleeping habits also affect your back.

4

WHAT IS GOOD POSTURE?

Posture is the single most important factor in determining the health of your back. Poor posture is the main cause of back problems. It leads to early, often irreversible, degeneration of the bones and joints of the spine, it causes muscular imbalance and tension, and it creates loose or over-taut ligaments – all of which result in back pain. The best way to look after your back, therefore, is to learn correct posture and then to maintain it in any activity you undertake. Learning correct posture can be difficult. We become so accustomed to the posture that we habitually adopt that attempts to correct it seem unnatural: good posture actually feels wrong and uncomfortable to begin with, or even lopsided. Posture can only be corrected over an extended period of time. We all have a tendency to slip back into our old ways, and remembering to maintain the correct stance during everyday routine activities requires a conscious effort.

RECOGNIZING POOR STANDING POSTURE

There are two common standing postures that are harmful to the back. Both of them place an unnatural burden on the spinal muscles, which can never fully relax and as a result become tense and painful. The ligaments are put under stress and, over time, the spinal joints will be affected. The first of these postures, the slouch, is readily recognized as unhealthy by most people. It is shown on the near right. The other type of posture, the "soldier's stance" (far right), is the opposite of this and is sometimes mistakenly regarded as desirable, but it is in fact just as damaging to the spine.

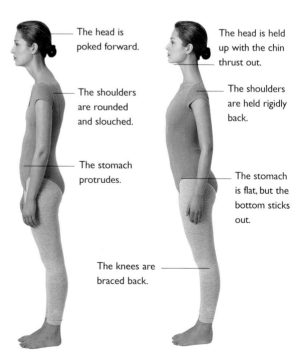

The head is poked forward.

The shoulders are rounded and slouched.

The stomach protrudes.

The head is held up with the chin thrust out.

The shoulders are held rigidly back.

The stomach is flat, but the bottom sticks out.

The knees are braced back.

RECOGNIZING GOOD STANDING POSTURE

Good posture means holding your body in such a way that each joint bears an equal share of the pressure on the spine and the pressure is evenly applied across the surfaces of the joints. The muscles should be relaxed with just enough tension in them to maintain the position, and the spine should curve naturally and gracefully – neither flat nor arched. To check your posture when standing, stand in front of a full-length mirror wearing only your underwear.

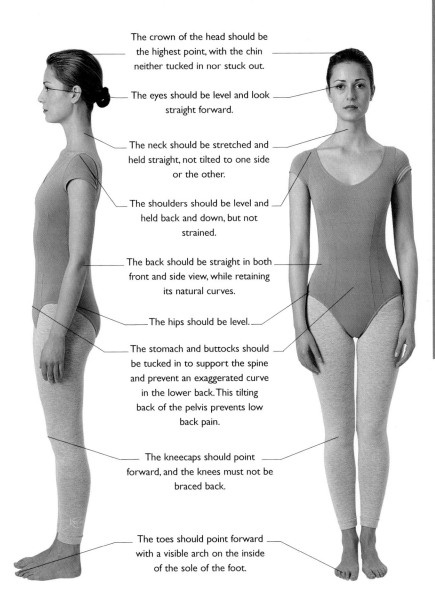

The crown of the head should be the highest point, with the chin neither tucked in nor stuck out.

The eyes should be level and look straight forward.

The neck should be stretched and held straight, not tilted to one side or the other.

The shoulders should be level and held back and down, but not strained.

The back should be straight in both front and side view, while retaining its natural curves.

The hips should be level.

The stomach and buttocks should be tucked in to support the spine and prevent an exaggerated curve in the lower back. This tilting back of the pelvis prevents low back pain.

The kneecaps should point forward, and the knees must not be braced back.

The toes should point forward with a visible arch on the inside of the sole of the foot.

4

IMPROVING POSTURE

With time and effort, bad postural habits can be gradually eliminated, and eventually the correct posture comes to feel right. Try the exercises below or use the Alexander Technique (see page 108) to correct poor posture so your movements become fluid and effortless, thereby relieving strain on your back.

EXERCISES TO CORRECT YOUR POSTURE

■ Stand in front of a mirror in your underwear. Start with the feet exercises and work up the body, maintaining the correct positions as you work from your feet to your neck and head.

■ Stand with your feet hip width apart, with the toes pointing forward. The weight of the body should be evenly distributed between the two feet and between the heel and ball of each foot.

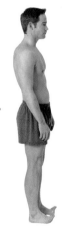
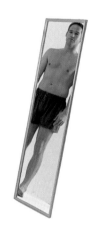

FEET

1 Sway backward slightly and feel your weight passing through your heels. Sway forward and feel the weight passing through the balls of your feet.

2 Raise your toes only off the ground and feel your weight balanced evenly between the balls and heels of the feet; then lower the toes.

4

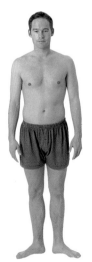

HIPS

1 Tilt the hips back and forth (see the pelvic tilt exercise on page 57). Repeat three times and then hold when the pelvis is tucked under in the correct neutral position. Tighten your stomach muscles hard, breathing out at the same time. Repeat a few times and then relax them slightly, keeping the stomach held in.

2 Turn your legs so your knees and toes are pointing out. Then point them in. Finally return to the neutral position with the knees and toes facing forward. Repeat three times.

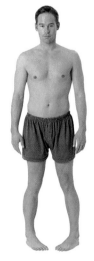

CHEST

I Breathe in deeply, moving your chest up and out and your shoulders down and back. Hold for a count of three and exhale, relaxing the shoulder and chest muscles. Repeat three times and then hold in the exhaled position.

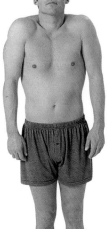

2 Hunch your shoulders up hard, hold for a count of three and let them go.

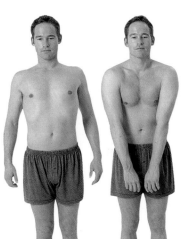

3 Pull your shoulders back so your shoulder blades are pulled together.

4 Then pull the shoulders forward to round the back. Repeat, ending with the shoulder blades pulled together. Relax the muscles and let your shoulders settle back and down.

NECK AND HEAD

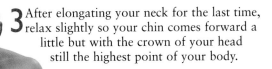

I Elongate your neck pulling your chin in at the same time. Feel your neck stretching, as though someone is pulling you up by the hair at the crown of your head.

2 Let your head fall back with your chin stuck up and out. Alternate this with the neck stretch exercise (step 1) three times.

3 After elongating your neck for the last time, relax slightly so your chin comes forward a little but with the crown of your head still the highest point of your body.

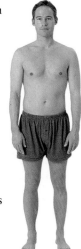

4 Finally, check that the position of the rest of your body is still correct; hold the posture for a few minutes and then continue with your normal activities. Try to repeat this series of checks a few times each day, concentrating on correcting any personal faults. Maintain the position while walking around as well as when standing still, and it will soon become a habit.

4

HOW TO SIT

Sitting puts up to two-and-a-half times more stress on the lower spine than standing, so people who spend a large part of their day sitting are particularly vulnerable to backache and long-term back problems. Leaning forward increases the stress even more. It is vital, therefore, that you sit correctly, with the spine straight and upright rather than slouched, so that the body's weight is evenly distributed down to the hips and pelvis.

THE CORRECT SEATING ANGLE

Ideally, the seat of the chair will slant downward, at an angle of about five degrees, so that the weight can be further transferred from the hips down the thighs and knees to the floor. There are various "back" chairs and wedged pillows on the market, both for home and office use, but these tend to be expensive, and it is usually possible to learn correct sitting posture using your own chairs and a few accessories.

4

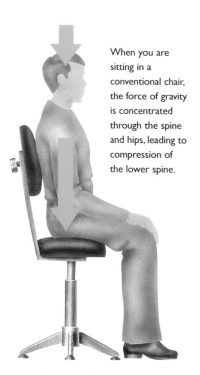

When you are sitting in a conventional chair, the force of gravity is concentrated through the spine and hips, leading to compression of the lower spine.

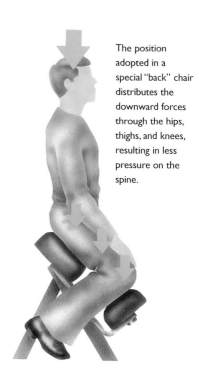

The position adopted in a special "back" chair distributes the downward forces through the hips, thighs, and knees, resulting in less pressure on the spine.

Conventional sitting posture

Sitting posture in a "back" chair

CORRECT SITTING POSTURE

- Sit well back in the chair with your weight on the buttocks and thighs, not the top of the buttocks and sacrum.

- Your thighs should be level with the ground. The knees should be level with, or slightly lower than, the thighs, and the lower legs should be at right angles to the feet. The legs should not be crossed – never sit with your legs crossed for a long period of time as it twists the spine. If you have to cross your legs, regularly alternate which leg is crossed over the other.

- Your feet should be planted on the ground and not dangling – keep them hip width apart if the situation allows.

- Your back must be straight, with support for the lower back – a lumbar roll, a small oblong pillow, or a rolled-up towel wedged in the small of the back are effective if the chair has no built-in support.

- Your shoulders should be down, back, and relaxed. Shoulder support is relaxing but not vital.

- Keep your head held straight and level, not poked forward.

THINGS TO AVOID

- Soft chairs – put a plank or board under the seat.

- Bucket chairs – their rounded shape encourages the lumbar spine to flex.

- Deep chairs where you cannot sit back fully and have your lower legs and feet at right angles.

- Chairs that are too high or too low so that the feet cannot reach the ground or the thighs are higher than the hips. Low chairs may put extra strain on the back when you get out of the chair.

- Having the television in a position that makes you look down to watch it, or having the volume so low that you have to crane forward to hear it.

- Holding a book, magazine, or newspaper in such a way that you have to look down to read it. Hold it well up or place it on some pillows on your lap.

- Sitting for long periods of time. Every 30 minutes or so, stand up and arch backward three times and move around, releasing any tension in the back. Commercial breaks are good reminders to move when watching television. Remember to do a few pelvic tilts (see pages 56-57) when sitting for any length of time, especially if you cannot get up.

4

BACK CARE AT WORK

The sedentary lifestyle that modern office work imposes on many of us is potentially harmful to our backs. The design and positioning of your office furniture, and the maintenance of correct sitting posture, are therefore of considerable importance. Modern office furniture is designed to reduce the risk of back problems, but not all companies can afford the latest ergonomic designs, and those who work from home may have to make do with the furniture already available. Whatever the circumstances, you should try to organize your seating arrangements in such a way as to minimize the strain on your back.

GENERAL MEASURES

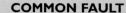

■ If you have to spend long periods leaning over a desk drawing or reading, try to obtain a sloping work surface or drawing board of the type used by designers and draftsmen.

■ If possible, vary your tasks during the day so you do not spend too long doing any one thing.

■ If you spend long periods of time sitting during the working day, balance this by doing some exercise before and after work. Do some stretches when you first get up (see pages 46-51), try to walk at least part of the way to and from work, or go for a short brisk walk upon your return in the evening.

4

COMMON FAULT

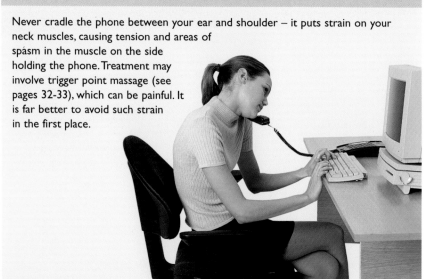

Never cradle the phone between your ear and shoulder – it puts strain on your neck muscles, causing tension and areas of spasm in the muscle on the side holding the phone. Treatment may involve trigger point massage (see pages 32-33), which can be painful. It is far better to avoid such strain in the first place.

WORKING AT A DESKTOP

There is no one chair that suits everyone, so your office chair needs to be adjustable in seat height, seat angle, and the position of the back rest. Even if you feel supported and comfortable while sitting, take frequent breaks, get up, move around, and stretch your spine back five or six times to counteract any flattening or pressure on the lower back.

■ The back of the chair should be upright but slightly molded, or have a back rest to support the lumbar curve of the lower back, and it should be tall enough to support the full width of your shoulders.

■ If you have been typing continuously for more than half an hour, stop and wriggle your fingers and rotate the wrists in both directions to ease any tension in the muscles and tendons of the forearms.

■ The center of your computer screen should be level with your eyes so you do not have to look down to read it, thereby straining the neck and upper back muscles. If you cannot raise the screen with a block or a thick book, angle it upward.

■ The seat should be at a height that allows the feet to be planted on the ground with the lower legs positioned vertically above them.

■ The seat should be deep enough to support the full length of the thighs.

■ The chair seat should be horizontal or tilted forward by about five degrees.

■ The forearms should be held just below horizontal so your fingers can touch the keyboard without the wrist being arched backward.

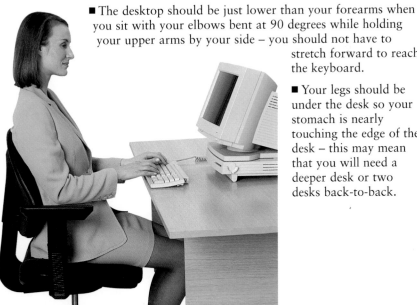

■ The desktop should be just lower than your forearms when you sit with your elbows bent at 90 degrees while holding your upper arms by your side – you should not have to stretch forward to reach the keyboard.

4

■ Your legs should be under the desk so your stomach is nearly touching the edge of the desk – this may mean that you will need a deeper desk or two desks back-to-back.

HOW TO LIFT CORRECTLY

More people injure their backs through lifting than in any other way. People tend to lift things up – or put them down – using the relatively weak back muscles rather than the strong leg muscles. You should use your whole body when you lift something, not just your arms and back, and lifting should be balanced and controlled, not a jerky heaving movement. Picking up even a light object incorrectly can also damage the back if it proves to be the last straw for a spine that is already strained.

CAUSES OF PROBLEMS WHEN LIFTING

Lifting is most likely to cause problems when the back has already been damaged in some way or other. Weakness in muscles and ligaments, muscular tension or imbalance, and degeneration of the spine (osteoarthritis) are all potential sources of back pain when lifting. Immediate causes include:

■ Twisting while lifting – even if the object is only a letter or handbag.

■ Lifting something of an unexpected weight.

■ Using a wrong lifting technique.

■ Lifting something at your side rather than in front of you.

■ Carrying or picking up a load away from the body, for example, unloading bags from the trunk. A weight carried away from the body puts ten times the stress on the spine as the same weight carried held into the body.

■ Carrying a heavy load on one side of the body.

4

TIPS FOR TROUBLE-FREE LIFTING

■ To carry a heavy weight, hug it to the center of your body and keep your back straight with the pelvis tucked in.

■ Never carry a heavy load on one side of the body: divide it if at all possible into two loads of equal weight.

■ To put an object down, reverse the procedure for lifting, squatting down with one leg in front of the other and with a straight back.

■ Be careful to stand up correctly once you have put an object down since your spine will be vulnerable to damage by any twisting or jerking movement.

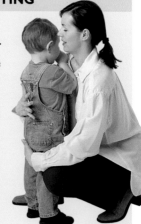

CORRECT LIFTING TECHNIQUE

1 Check the weight of the object to be lifted – is it light or heavy?

2 Stand as close as possible to the object with your feet on either side of it rather than behind or to one side.

3 Position one foot in front of the other so that you are well-balanced.

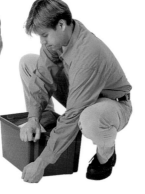

4 Use your hip and knee joints to squat down, keeping your back straight, until the object is between your legs.

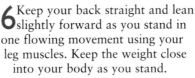

5 Place one hand completely beneath the load and grasp or hold it firmly with the other. If the object is very heavy or an awkward shape, lift one edge up slightly to get your hand underneath.

6 Keep your back straight and lean slightly forward as you stand in one flowing movement using your leg muscles. Keep the weight close into your body as you stand.

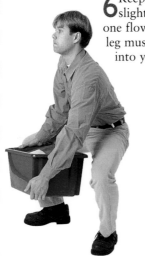

7 Never lift and twist at the same time: lift until you are standing upright and then turn the whole body around to the direction in which you want to go.

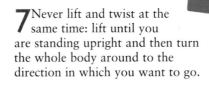

4

IN THE YARD

The yard is a danger zone for those with bad backs as well as for those who are simply out of condition. Gardening involves much crouching, bending, lifting, carrying, and other activities that put considerable stress on the back. Also, people have a tendency to do one type of work in the yard, be it pruning, digging, mowing, or weeding, for several hours at a stretch. The fact that many people garden in irregular spurts rather than on a routine basis can make matters worse. As a result, it is hardly surprising that the yard is the most common place for back problems to occur, and you should make care of your back one of your highest gardening priorities.

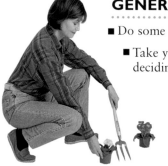

GENERAL PRECAUTIONS

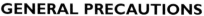

■ Do some gentle stretches before you start gardening.

■ Take your general state of fitness into account when deciding how long you will garden.

■ Observe the basic rules of lifting: bend your knees, not your back, at all times.

■ Work should be taken slowly with frequent rests and back stretches.

■ Do not dig when the ground is wet or hard.

■ Do not try to dig a whole bed at once, but change to weeding, planting, or pruning for a while after finishing a section.

■ Buy the long-handled tools and special spades that are now made for people with bad backs.

■ Kneel on a gardening mat to plant or weed and get as close as possible to where you are working.

■ Take care when pruning high branches; even light tools can strain the back when held high.

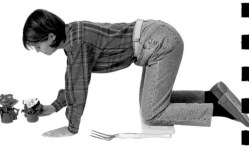

■ Use a hose rather than a watering can wherever possible, but if you have to use a watering can, only fill it half full.

■ Keep the tool shed neat and organized so you do not have to bend over things to get a tool.

■ Keep sacks of potting mixture and other materials in the shed and put small amounts at a time into a container.

4

DIGGING WITHOUT STRAIN

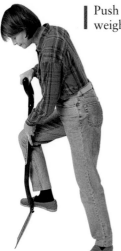

1 Push a spade in close to your front foot and use your body weight rather than your muscles to push it into the ground.

2 Crouch and grasp the handle near the blade, lever out the earth, and without lifting it high, turn the blade over and drop the soil back. Do not attempt to turn or shovel too much earth at one time; the job might take longer to complete, but you are less likely to injure your back if you shovel only small amounts at a time.

WHEELBARROWS

Wheelbarrows are dangerous tools for those with a chronic back problem. The act of lifting a weight in front of you and then pushing at the same time puts enormous pressure on the spine.

■ Make sure your wheelbarrow is light and well-designed so the weight of the load is carried over the wheel, not near the handles.

■ Only use a wheelbarrow over even, hard ground where you are not trying to prevent it from twisting sideways at the same time.

■ Only use a wheelbarrow when you must; many things, like weeds, can be put on a groundsheet or put straight into refuse bags.

MOWERS

If you have a lawn and a back problem, you should have a motorized lawn mower. Avoid lifting a heavy mower and take care on turns and bends. Rotary or cylinder models are the best.

■ Stand close to the mower and adjust the handles so you do not have to bend forward.

■ Keep the mower well serviced so it starts easily, especially if it has a pull-cord to start the engine.

■ If you have to use a manual mower, push it, don't pull it, since pushing puts less strain on the back.

WEIGHT AND THE BACK

There is no doubt that being overweight has an adverse effect on the back. Excess fat has no beneficial effects on the body. Unlike muscle, which protects and supports the joints and relieves them of pressure, fat merely increases the load that the joints have to bear. This particularly affects the weight-bearing joints, especially in the lower back and hip. Not only does the additional stress increase the general wear and tear on the joints, leading to the early onset of osteoarthritis, but it also makes the back more vulnerable to a variety of other ailments, including strained ligaments and disk problems.

HOW WEIGHT AFFECTS THE BACK

Overweight people, particularly men, tend to carry much of their extra weight in their stomachs. This weakens the stomach muscles, making it difficult for them to support the spine. Without good muscular control, the spine is much more vulnerable. The abdominal muscles also support the spine during any strenuous activity, such as lifting or carrying. When tense, the abdominals increase the pressure within the abdominal cavity, so the cavity itself can take some of the weight-bearing role, and this relieves the stress on the spine.

ARE YOU THE CORRECT WEIGHT?

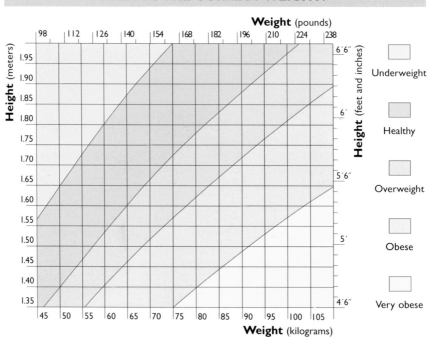

4

EFFECTS ON THE SPINE OF BEING OVERWEIGHT

■ Poor posture – an increased lordosis, or hollow in the small of the back – so that the weight is not borne centrally by the disks and vertebrae.

■ Early onset of osteoarthritis due to excessive load bearing.

■ Flattened disks that are prone to prolapse – a "slipped disk" – and which also lose their ability to act as shock absorbers.

■ Facet joints between the vertebrae become too tight because the thinner disks mean that the articulating surfaces are squashed too closely together. There is increased friction in the joint with any movement so that the joints are liable to become inflamed and painful.

■ Wear on the spine, together with weak abdominal muscles, makes the back an inadequate scaffold for lifting, increasing the likelihood of acute back problems when doing so.

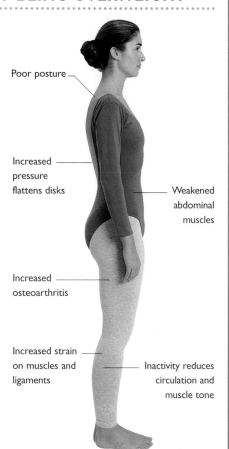

Poor posture

Increased pressure flattens disks

Weakened abdominal muscles

Increased osteoarthritis

Increased strain on muscles and ligaments

Inactivity reduces circulation and muscle tone

4

YOUR BODY TYPE AND YOUR BACK

There is some controversy over whether certain physical shapes are more prone to back problems than others. However, with two possible exceptions, it appears that body type is not significant; weight and posture are considerably more important.

■ Tall males, whether thin or overweight, appear to show a tendency to suffer more back problems than those of average or short stature. However, this is more likely to be because of poor posture, due to constant stooping than a direct consequence of height.

■ Similarly, large-breasted women have a slightly greater incidence of back problems. Again, this is more likely to be postural than inherent, since women with large breasts often hunch their shoulders to disguise the fact.

DIET AND WEIGHT

If you suffer from a back problem and are overweight, it is vital that you reduce your weight to within the recommended range through sensible eating and exercise. The food we eat provides the energy for all the functions of the body. The metabolic rate is the speed with which the body uses up this energy. Weight control is mainly a question of balancing the energy input – the food we eat – and the energy output – the energy used in muscular activity and body maintenance. If more energy is taken in than is required by the body, the excess is stored in the form of fat and weight increases. If less is taken in than required, then the body makes up the energy deficiency by utilizing the stored fat and weight is lost.

LOSING WEIGHT

■ Aim to lose no more than 2 pounds a week.

■ Change the balance of your diet if necessary. The best slimming diets are based on a high intake of unrefined carbohydrates, moderate protein intake, and low fat intake.

■ Check your calorie intake. The average daily calorie requirement ranges from 1,900 for a woman to around 2,350 for a man, although individuals may differ according to their level of physical activity. You should never let your calorie intake fall below 1,000 to 1,500 calories a day.

■ Do not try crash dieting: the body responds to starvation by slowing down the metabolic rate, so less food is required for it to function. Such diets can lead to severe malnourishment and muscle wasting.

■ Adopt sensible eating habits. It is better to eat little and often – four or five times a day if possible – than to have just one or two large meals a day.

■ If you do find yourself craving food between meals, often mid-morning or mid-afternoon, restore your blood sugar levels by eating something containing complex (unrefined) carbohydrates, such as a slice of wholewheat bread or a banana, rather than a piece of cake or a candy bar.

■ Serve your food on smaller plates – portions won't look any smaller than they did before – and avoid snacking by eating only at the table.

■ Be wary of slimming pills and "miracle" cures. Check with your doctor before taking any type of slimming aid, particularly if you are taking other medication.

■ Many people find that joining a diet group, for example Weightwatchers, can be a great help in sticking to a slimming program.

■ Remember that exercise, especially aerobic exercise such as brisk walking, is a vital part of any attempt at weight loss since it raises the metabolic rate.

4

HINTS FOR HEALTHY EATING.

- Cut down on fats – remember that red meats contain a high percentage of invisible fat.

- Reduce your intake of sugar.

- Cut down on refined and processed foods.

- Reduce your alcohol intake – alcohol has a high caloric content.

- Cut down on your intake of caffeine, found in coffee, tea, and soft drinks.

- Check the food label on low-fat or low-sugar items since one often has a high content of the other.

- Eat wholegrain foods and make sure you have an adequate fiber intake.

- Eat at least three servings of vegetables a day. Do not overcook.

- Eat plenty of fish, especially oily fish.

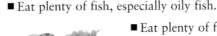

- Eat plenty of fresh fruit.

- Drink at least 8 cups of water a day.

PRECAUTIONS

Dieting unwisely can be as harmful as unhealthy eating. Plan to lose weight gradually, not overnight.

- If you feel the urge to carry on dieting after you have reached your recommended weight, consult your doctor. There is a possibility that this urge may develop into anorexia nervosa or bulimia, both of which are serious conditions requiring medical help.

- Don't attempt to lose weight too quickly. The body may have adequate fat reserves to provide energy, but there are many other essential ingredients in food, and depriving the body of these can have serious consequences.

- In rare cases, weight problems are caused by a disorder of the pituitary or thyroid gland, or the pancreas. If you have serious difficulty in keeping your weight down, you should consult your doctor.

OTHER HEALTH BENEFITS

Losing excess weight does not just help your back. Reducing the percentage of body fat lessens your chances of developing many other serious health problems, including:

- Heart attacks.

- Strokes.

- High blood pressure.

- Diabetes.

- Osteoarthritis.

- Kidney and gallstone problems.

4

RELAXATION AND SLEEP

People with back pain often find it difficult to relax and get adequate rest and sleep. Pain causes muscles to spasm, and a muscle in spasm is painful, so a vicious circle sets in. It is also easy to worry about a back problem, and anxiety stimulates the body's "fight or flight" response. This instinctive response to a threat – whether real or imagined – was vital in our ancestors' day, but it is less useful now. However, our bodies have not changed and still prepare for action. The heart beats faster, breathing becomes rapid, and the muscles become tense, but all to no avail if the tension is not then released by furious activity. In time, unless you take positive steps to learn how to relax, you are likely to suffer from chronic stress. The stress increases muscle spasm, lessens the flexibility of the ligaments, and increases your awareness of pain; you have become trapped in a vicious circle.

SEVEN STEPS TO RELAXATION

Different relaxation techniques work best for different people. Find one which works well for you – be it massage, meditation, or visualization therapy – or follow the instructions below. Exercise before a rest helps you to relax more fully, as the release of endorphins during exercise reduces any pain.

1 Wearing loose, comfortable clothes, lie down on a mat or bed in a dimly lit room. Place a pillow under your knees to take any strain off your back and one under your head if you wish. Make sure you will be undisturbed.

2 Empty your mind and take three deep breaths through your nose, emptying your lungs each time you breathe out. Relax.

3 Tense the muscles of one leg. Hold for a count of five and release. Repeat three times and then repeat with the other leg.

4 Tighten your buttock muscles, hold for a count of five and release. Tense your stomach muscles, hold for a count of five and release.

5 Tense one arm, clenching the fingers into a fist. Hold for a count of five and repeat three times. Repeat with the other arm.

6 Hunch your shoulders up hard toward your head; hold and relax. Repeat three times. Tighten your face up into a grimace; hold and release.

7 Tense your whole body three times and then relax. Breathe deeply and slowly and feel your body sinking down. Keeping your mind empty, breathe naturally, and slide into a semi-sleep.

SLEEP

Sleep is as important as
relaxation for the
human body, though
the amount of sleep
required differs from one
person to another and
varies with lifestyle, health,
and age. If you are suffering
from an attack of back pain,
it is important to get enough
sleep so the damaged tissues
can heal and the spine can have a
rest from its weight-bearing role. A
comfortable and supportive bed is vital

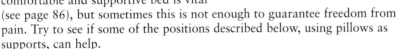

(see page 86), but sometimes this is not enough to guarantee freedom from
pain. Try to see if some of the positions described below, using pillows as
supports, can help.

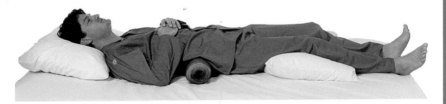

■ If you are lying on your back, place a pillow under your knees to take any
strain off the spine.

■ Try placing a heating pad or well-covered hot-water bottle under your
back – the warmth will help to relax the muscles.

■ Use only one pillow under your head – your neck should be in a straight line
with the rest of the spine.

■ If you sleep on your side, place a pillow between your knees to prevent your
hip from rolling forward and try a bolster up against your chest.

■ Place a small pillow in the arch formed by your waist.

■ If you are lying on your stomach, place a pillow under your feet and another
under your abdomen.

4

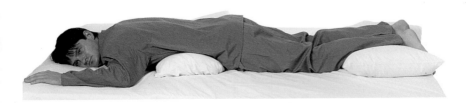

CHOOSING A BED

Your bed and mattress should last for a good few years, so it is important to buy one that is suitable for your back – whether you have a problem at the moment or not. The word "orthopedic" when used to describe a bed does not necessarily mean that it is the best type for a bad back – though it does usually mean that it will be more expensive. In general, most people with back problems find that a mattress with independent springs on a firm base suits them best. But it is essential to test any bed before buying it. Any good bed salesperson will encourage you to stay and try the bed out for as long as you like.

■ Lie on the bed in the position in which you normally sleep, and stay there for long enough to be sure that you are comfortable.

■ Check that the mattress allows you to change position easily. Most people move around a fair amount in their sleep, and it is important that you are able to do so. If you stay in the same position for too long, some ligaments become over-stretched and lose their ability to support the spine.

■ If you have a partner of greatly different height or weight, test the bed together. A bed with a pair of mattresses of different degrees of firmness may be the best solution.

■ The base of the bed should be firm or slatted – avoid bases that are soft or springy since they will decrease the life of your mattress.

■ Check that the bed is of a suitable height for you – it should be easy to get in and out of it

■ When choosing bedding, remember that bedding that is too tight will restrict movement, so if you have not previously done so, try a comforter.

Too soft

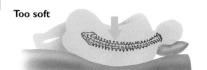

A mattress that is too soft encourages the middle of the spine to sag and makes it difficult to move freely during the night.

Too hard

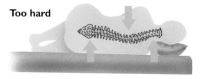

A mattress that is too hard does not give at the hips and shoulders and therefore may distort the spine.

Correct

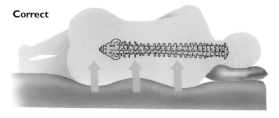

A mattress that is correct for your needs is firm enough to support your weight without sagging, but allows some "give" at the hips and shoulders while supporting the spine and making it easy to turn and move.

SPECIAL CONDITIONS

This chapter deals with some of the special conditions that can affect your back, such as pregnancy, which puts extra demands on it. Many terms frequently used to describe back problems are precisely defined here, in order to dispel some commonly held misunderstandings. Osteoarthritis, for example, is not a disease, but a natural part of the aging process – but one which can, however, be delayed, depending on how well you look after your body in general and your back in particular. Sciatica, too, is not a disease in itself but a collection of symptoms with a number of different causes. On the following pages you will find out how you can avoid a variety of specific problems and/or relieve the pain they cause.

5

PREGNANCY

The last few months of pregnancy can be a particularly difficult time for women who have back problems. Even women who have never experienced back pain before are likely to notice aches in their lower back, particularly after standing for long periods.

WHY PREGNANCY AFFECTS THE BACK

One of the main reasons for back pain in pregnancy is that the body prepares itself for birth by producing a hormone called relaxin. This hormone relaxes the ligaments that support the sacroiliac joint – where the spine joins the pelvis – to increase the size of the birth canal through which the baby will pass during labor. Unfortunately, relaxin affects other ligaments, too, with the result that any twisting or bending is not supported or restrained in the usual way. This normally only gives rise to aches and pain, but there is a possibility that damage will be caused to the lower back – especially in those who suffer from back problems.

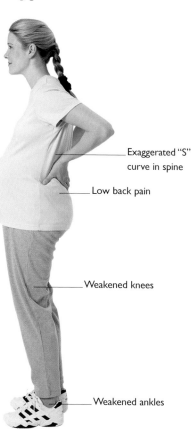

Exaggerated "S" curve in spine

Low back pain

Weakened knees

Weakened ankles

5

SPECIAL PROBLEMS OF MID-PREGNANCY

You may feel an intense pain all over your lower back, and often also in the groin, if you twist your spine during the middle months of pregnancy – as when stretching behind you or rolling over in bed. The reason for this is that the rotation of the spine causes the sacroiliac joint, whose ligaments have already been relaxed by hormones, to open and close slightly, producing the pain. Avoid any such activity if you can, but do not worry that the problem is permanent. It normally clears up after the sixth month, when the baby tips farther forward and is not resting against the spine in the same way.

YOUR CHANGING CENTER OF GRAVITY

The effect of relaxin on the ligaments is compounded by another factor unique to pregnancy. During the later stages, a pregnant woman carries a considerable amount of extra weight at her front. This moves her center of gravity forward with the result that the back muscles have to work harder to maintain an upright position. In response, the pelvis tends to tilt forward, exaggerating the lumbar curve of the spine. This, in turn, means that the vertebrae are out of alignment, and this puts strain on the facet joints. To complete the vicious circle, the strain on the facet joints puts more stress on the ligaments, which are already weaker. The result can be anything from a dull, constant ache to inflammation and sciatica (see pages 98-99).

PROTECTIVE MEASURES

There are a number of things that you can do to reduce the chances that a problem will develop:

■ Take special care to maintain correct posture (see pages 68-71) throughout pregnancy.

■ Practice pelvic tilts as often as you can (see page 27) – until they become second nature.

■ Lift and bend correctly (see pages 76-77).

■ Exercise to keep your muscles strong and flexible (see pages 48-55), which will maximize support to the spine, so you can bear the extra weight of pregnancy.

■ Do not wear high-heeled shoes, since they throw the body off balance and exaggerate the lumbar curve – even before the threat to the lumbar spine that comes with pregnancy.

■ Avoid staying in the same position for too long; doing so over-stretches the ligaments, which are already relaxed.

■ Minimize the necessity to bend by altering the height of work surfaces (see pages 62-63).

■ Do the special back exercises for pregnancy shown in the next two pages.

5

Warning

Consult your doctor if pain that started in the back starts to run down your leg: you may have a disk prolapse and sciatica (see page 98). Back pain that comes on suddenly in late pregnancy may in some cases be the first sign of the start of labor. Call your doctor.

EXERCISES IN PREGNANCY

The best way of preventing back pain during pregnancy is to do the exercises shown below on a daily basis. This is especially important if you have previously suffered from back problems, since pregnancy not only puts an extra physical stress on your back but, as a result of hormonal changes, reduces the effectiveness of the ligaments that help resist extra stresses at other times.

EXERCISES FOR PREVENTION AND TREATMENT

Warm up gently before doing these exercises. Adapt the routine on pages 46-47. Omit step 8 and do the walking in place (step 9) gently with only moderate leg lifts. Aim to repeat the exercises below five times, morning and night, but make sure that you do not overdo things. It may take some time for you to build up to five repetitions.

KNEE ROLLS AND CAT ARCHES

Do the knee rolls described on page 57 and back arching exercise on page 49 (steps 3 and 4). Be sure to discontinue any exercise that causes discomfort or pain. Only do as many repetitions as you can manage with ease.

KNEE BENDS

1 Stand upright, holding onto a bar or the back of a chair for support, with your feet wide apart and your toes pointing out.

2 Bend your knees, going down as far as you can before returning to the upright position. Remember to keep your back straight. Practice this throughout your pregnancy so that you can eventually get down into the squatting position and rest in it comfortably.

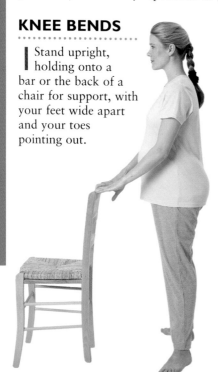

5

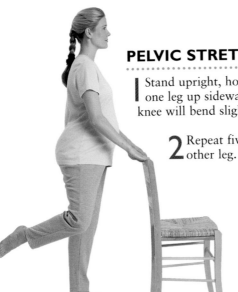

PELVIC STRETCHES

1 Stand upright, holding the back of a chair. Lift one leg up sideways and slightly back – your knee will bend slightly. Repeat five times.

2 Repeat five more times, using the other leg.

Warning

During this exercise you will feel a stretch along the thigh, your buttocks will tighten, and the pelvis will open slightly. This is normal.

BACK TWISTS

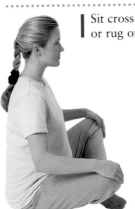

1 Sit cross-legged on an exercise mat or rug on the floor.

2 Place one hand on the floor behind you. Twist one side of your body so that you are looking over your shoulder in the same direction. Repeat, twisting the other side of the body.

RESTING TO EASE THE PAIN

Sometimes back pain during pregnancy is caused by the baby pushing up against the sciatic nerve. You may not know whether this is true in your case, but it is worth trying the following technique anyway – it is often effective at relieving pain. Rest for a few minutes while lying on your back with your knees bent at right angles and your lower legs at right angles to your thighs, resting them on pillows, a chair, or a stool. This is known as the psoas position.

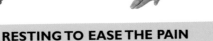

5

POSTNATAL EXERCISES

Keeping your back fit during pregnancy is only half the battle when you are having a baby. After the delivery you have more work to do, not only to get your figure back but to recondition the muscles and ligaments that have been affected by your extra weight and the physical pressures exerted during your baby's delivery. The exercises shown below will help return your joints, muscles, and ligaments – and so your back as a whole – to full working order.

RESTORING THE TISSUES

The nine months of increasing weight and the forces exerted during the delivery itself combine to make your stomach muscles very weak after the birth of your baby. In fact, the paired abdominal muscles separate slightly during late pregnancy. The result is that the abdominal muscles can play little part in supporting the spine. The ligaments that support the lower back and pelvis have also been stretched and weakened. It is important, therefore, that both the muscles and the ligaments are strengthened so that the spine is supported properly. These exercises are designed to do this. Check with your doctor when it is safe to start exercising after the birth. Do as many repetitions as you can without strain, morning and night, building up over time to five repetitions of each exercise. Start your program with the pelvic tilts described on page 27.

STOMACH STRENGTHENERS

1 Lie on the floor with your knees bent and your feet on the floor.

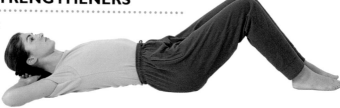

2 Use your stomach muscles to lift your head and shoulders up toward your knees. Do not strain – you will gradually be able to increase the distance you can lift them as your stomach muscles regain their strength and alignment.

5

STANDING BENDS

1 Raise your arms above your head in a star shape, then bend forward – first toward your knees; and then down toward the ground. Rise carefully, making sure you uncurl your back. Do not bounce.

2 Stand with your legs wide apart and bend one arm as far down its side as it will go; repeat with the other arm.

TWO BY TWOS

1 Kneel on all fours with the hip and shoulder joints at right angles. Bring one knee in toward the chest.

2 Then stretch the leg out behind you. Lower the leg and repeat with the other leg.

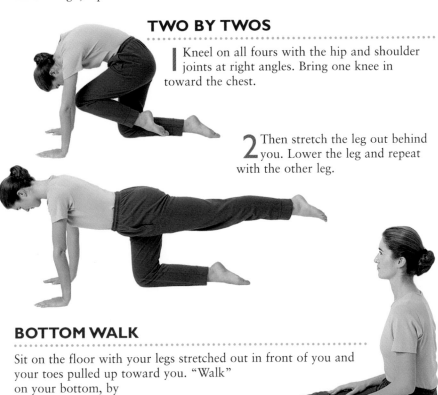

BOTTOM WALK

Sit on the floor with your legs stretched out in front of you and your toes pulled up toward you. "Walk" on your bottom, by pushing one leg forward and then the other.

5

Warning

Do not attempt these exercises if you had a cesarean section, a forceps delivery, or other difficult birth; special postnatal exercises will be prescribed for you by medical staff in such cases. Even if you had a normal delivery, take great care not to strain at any time, because doing so can make the abdominal muscles separate farther. Start your exercise program very gently, and build up the intensity of the exercises and the number of repetitions slowly.

OSTEOARTHRITIS

To a certain extent, osteoarthritis is inevitable. It is not a disease but a term used to describe the degenerative damage to cartilage and bone that is a natural part of the process of aging. There are several risk factors that make the early onset of osteoarthritis more likely, but there is also a range of preventive measures that can help delay its onset. Both of these depend on the use and abuse of exercise and the importance of looking after your body.

RISK FACTORS

■ Inadequate exercise. Cartilage in joints is lubricated by fluid, but the production of this fluid is reduced if the joints are not moved adequately, increasing friction.

■ Excessive exercise. Repeated overuse of the joints increases the rate at which cartilage is worn away; it also makes minor wrenches and strains more likely.

■ Poor posture. Unnatural strains on the joints and the lack of muscular support, caused by poor posture, increase friction and wear.

■ Obesity. Excess weight increases the strains on the spine and, by altering the center of gravity, reduces the ability of the abdominal muscles to support the spine.

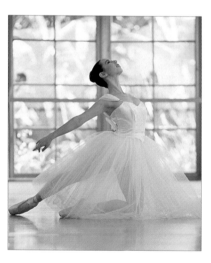

■ Poor lifting technique. Incorrect lifting causes tissue damage that redistributes stresses and strains, increasing friction.

■ A previous bone fracture. Again this distorts stresses, so increasing friction.

Ballet dancers, athletes, and others whose work involves strenuous physical training are particularly susceptible to the early onset of osteoarthritis.

5

HOW TO DELAY THE ONSET OF OSTEOARTHRITIS

Though a certain amount of osteoarthritis is inevitable with age, it can be held at bay, or at least controlled, by a program of moderate exercise and by avoidance of the risk factors. Do flexibility exercises (see pages 48-51) and make sure you put your spine through its full range of movements at least three times a week.

THE DEGENERATIVE PROCESS

The weight-bearing ends of articulating bones are covered with a smooth, tough cartilage called hyaline cartilage. In osteoarthritis, the areas of maximum contact are gradually worn away; as a result, other areas become brittle and fragmented so the bones grind over each other when any movement is made. In turn, this grinding wears away more cartilage. However, the spiral of damage has almost certainly begun some time before this, often as a result of minor stresses and strains that may not even have been noticed. A jarring movement or a wrench can tear some of the tissues around the vertebral joints and cause a tiny amount of bleeding. As these tears heal, they form scars, which have less "give," so the next minor wrench will tear other fibers – and so it goes on. The small muscles nearby go into a protective spasm to limit any movement and bind the joint close, but this increases the friction on the cartilage: the degenerative process has begun.

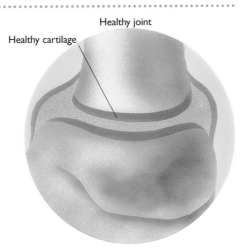

Healthy joint

Healthy cartilage

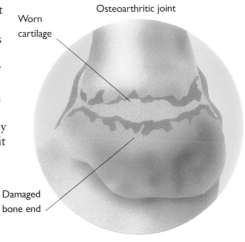

Osteoarthritic joint

Worn cartilage

Damaged bone end

BONE CHANGES

At the same time as the center of the cartilage is being worn away, the cartilage at the margins of the joint grows out into the joint space and starts to become bony – these bony spurs of former cartilage are known as osteophytes. Most people start to develop osteophytes around the main weight-bearing joints – the hips, the knees, and the lumbar vertebra – at around the age of 60, purely as a result of aging. Often they do not cause any problems apart from loss of range of movement and stiffness. However, in more advanced cases, when osteoarthritis has set in earlier in life due to one or other predisposing factors, the combination of eroded cartilages and osteophytes can cause severe pain and considerable difficulty with movement. In rare cases, osteophytes can compress spinal nerve roots or the spinal cord itself: this problem can only be treated by surgery (see pages 110-111).

5

OSTEOPOROSIS

Also known as brittle bone disease, osteoporosis is a condition in which the bones lose their calcium content and become thinner and less dense. As a result, they fracture easily. It affects all the bones of the body, but those of the spine, thigh, and forearm in particular. Like osteoarthritis, osteoporosis is to a certain extent part of the natural process of aging, and preventive measures can delay its onset in the majority of cases. Taking such measures is important, because once bone mass has been lost, it cannot be replaced – though research into new drugs holds promise that one day this will not be the case.

CAUSES OF OSTEOPOROSIS

It is possible for a person of either sex to develop osteoporosis at any age, but it is particularly prevalent in postmenopausal women. Causative factors include:

■ Menopause.

■ Early hysterectomy with one or both ovaries removed.

■ Long-term dieting, especially if dairy products are cut out.

■ Old age, since the body absorbs calcium less efficiently at this time.

■ Over-exercising – as in marathon running – which depletes the production of female hormones.

■ Low-calcium diet.

■ Inadequate weight-bearing exercise.

■ Bed rest.

■ High alcohol intake.

■ Heavy smoking.

■ Pregnancy – the growing baby takes calcium from the maternal bones if the mother's diet lacks this important mineral.

THE DISEASE PROCESS

Typically, by the age of 70, the average person has lost about a third of their bone density. Women are generally more severely affected than men. As far as the spine is concerned, osteoporosis affects the vertebral bodies – most often those of the thoracic spine, though sometimes the lumbar vertebrae are affected as well. As the condition develops, the bones of the vertebrae are compressed into a wedge shape, with the thinnest end of the wedge facing into the body. In the lumbar region this flattens the back, but in the thoracic area the result is pronounced kyphosis – an exaggerated outward bend of the spine that is sometimes known as a "dowager's hump" when seen in elderly women. Another effect of significant loss of bone density in the spine is that sufferers become shorter over time, sometimes by as much as 6 inches.

As the condition progresses, the density of the bone is gradually reduced to the point at which even minor pressure on the vertebrae, or relatively insignificant injury to them, can cause them to crumble and collapse – in advanced cases, merely the weight of the body pressing down on them is enough.

HOW OSTEOPOROSIS CAUSES PAIN

Osteoporosis is not painful in itself, but its effects can be very painful. The distortion of spinal curves causes tension and spasm in the spinal muscles, while a crushed or crumbling vertebra can trap the spinal column or spinal nerves, causing pain and immobility, and squash the facet joints together, causing inflammation.

HOW TO PREVENT OSTEOPOROSIS

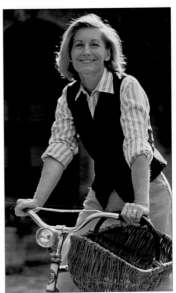

In rare cases, there is an early onset of osteoporosis that is not obviously linked to any obvious cause. However, most cases of the condition are linked to either a deficiency of calcium in the diet or a lack of the female hormone estrogen. This hormone has a preventive effect against osteoporosis, but when its production ceases after menopause, women's bones seem to absorb less calcium from the diet. If you have reason to suspect that you are at risk from osteoporosis, which tends to run in families, consult your doctor. He or she may suggest that you have a bone density scan to check whether the condition is present in your case. Otherwise, bear in mind these preventive measures, especially if you are a postmenopausal woman:

- Maintain a good level of vitamin D, which helps the calcium to be absorbed by the bones. A combined calcium and vitamin D supplement is convenient.

- Eat plenty of calcium-rich foods, such as milk, cheese, yogurt, sardines, herrings, spinach, nuts, red kidney beans, figs, apricots, sesame seeds, broccoli, and watercress. Low-fat dairy products contain as much calcium as full-fat varieties.

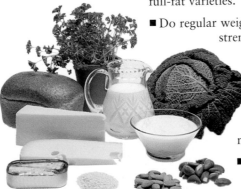

- Do regular weight-bearing exercise. Exercise strengthens the bones by laying down more calcium and other minerals.

- Correct your posture and learn how to lift correctly.

- Consider hormone replacement therapy after menopause.

- Reduce your intake of alcohol and stop smoking.

5

SCIATICA

The sciatic nerve, the longest nerve in the body, is made up of five or six spinal nerves that leave the spinal canal at the base of the spine and join up to form the one large nerve that runs down the leg. Sciatica is not, in fact, a medical condition, but a name for a set of symptoms that are caused by pressure on one or more of the elements of the sciatic nerve as it leaves the spine. The length of the nerve means that even though sciatica is a spinal problem, its effects may be felt a long way from the back.

CAUSES AND SYMPTOMS

The pressure on the sciatic nerve may arise from a prolapsed disk (see page 13), often called a slipped disk, or from the swelling around an inflamed facet joint. It can also become trapped as a result of osteoarthritic changes in the spine or, during pregnancy, be pressed against the spine by the extra weight of the fetus or by soft tissues that swell with water as a result of hormonal changes. On rare occasions, chronic sciatica can be caused by a fragment of disk cartilage that has broken off and is pressing on the sciatic nerve.

The symptoms of sciatica are unpleasant: an acute, shooting, unrelenting pain down the area of the body served by the part of the sciatic nerve that is trapped. Which area depends on which of the spinal nerves is pinched as they leave the spinal column. At its worst, the pain can start in the back and travel across the buttocks, into the hip, and down the back of the leg to the foot. There may also be pins and needles and, occasionally, numbness. In severe cases, in which sciatica lasts for a long time, the muscles supplied by the sciatic nerve may weaken.

CAUSES OF SCIATICA

A number of different factors can cause an attack of sciatica, but these are among the most common:

■ Poor posture.

■ Incorrect lifting technique.

■ Sudden, strenuous activity especially if you are unfit.

■ Sudden twisting movement without any muscular preparation.

■ Weak back and/or abdominal muscles.

■ Osteoarthritis.

■ Osteoporosis.

■ Pregnancy.

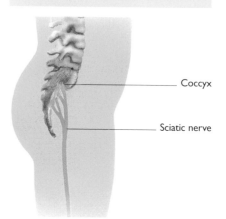

Coccyx

Sciatic nerve

5

DO'S AND DON'TS IN AN ATTACK

In most cases, an attack of sciatica resolves itself within a few weeks as the protruding disk is reabsorbed or the inflammation dies down. Sometimes, however, it can be caused by a condition that requires treatment by a specialist, so see your doctor if the pain does not start to diminish after a day and night of bed rest. Here are some do's and don'ts for the first 24 hours:

Do

■ Stop what you are doing immediately.

■ Try to lie down on your stomach with your hands by your side to relieve the pressure on the spine.

■ Go to bed for 24 hours (if you do not have a firm mattress, place a thin piece of wood beneath it).

■ Apply an ice pack to the small of your back. A bag of frozen peas is ideal, but cover it with a towel since ice can burn if it is placed directly onto the skin.

■ Take the recommended dose of painkillers – those incorporating an anti-inflammatory agent are best.

■ Relax and try not to worry about what you should be doing as tension will worsen the problem.

■ Crawl to the bathroom if walking upright is painful.

■ If the ice is no help, give yourself a heat rub or press a hot-water bottle, wrapped in a towel, to the area that is painful.

■ Remember what you were doing before the pain started.

■ Take note of which positions are comfortable and which are painful.

■ See a doctor if there is no improvement in 24 hours.

Don't

■ Don't ignore the pain: it is a sign of damage.

■ Don't bend, lift, twist, or carry anything.

■ Don't let anyone unqualified manipulate your back – a gentle massage avoiding the spine itself is all that anybody unqualified should attempt.

■ Don't return to normal activities once the attack is over without first strengthening your muscles and regaining flexibility (see pages 48-55).

■ Don't persist with any self-help measures that make your symptoms worse.

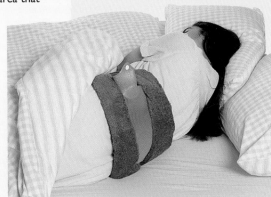

5

BENDS IN THE SPINE

The spine has four natural curves (see pages 10-11), which allow it to absorb the shock waves from the ground during walking and the stresses and strains caused by the body's weight and its movements. These natural curves can become distorted, either by disease or as a result of the demands placed on the muscles and joints by incorrect posture or a lack of adequate body maintenance over a period of time. The four main distortions of the spine's curves are discussed here.

SCOLIOSIS

Normally the spine runs straight down the back, but in scoliosis it is bent to one side. A serious scoliosis is sometimes present at birth, but it is often the result of one leg being shorter than the other: the spine is bent by the posture needed to accommodate this inequality. This type of scoliosis tends to develop in childhood and is treated by special braces, prescribed by an orthopedic surgeon, as well as by specialized exercises and, sometimes, surgery.

A less severe scoliosis may develop when someone who suffers from chronic back pain acquires the habit of leaning to one side to minimize the pain, or as the result of poor posture over time. Whatever its cause, a scoliosis shortens the muscles on one side of the body and makes them stiff. It becomes increasingly difficult to straighten the spine and the accumulation of the unequal stresses on it causes back pain, muscular tension, and a tendency to develop early osteoarthritis.

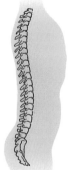

Normal spine
Back view

Normal spine
Side view

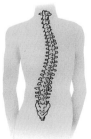

Scoliosis

COUNTERING SCOLIOSIS

■ Get the lengths of your legs checked and, if necessary, build up the heel in one shoe so that they are of equal length. A physical therapist can advise on this. In time the spine will straighten, though it may ache as it adapts to the correct position. Exercises will speed the process.

■ Treat the underlying back problem if the scoliosis has developed in an attempt to ease pain.

■ Maintain good posture (see pages 68-71).

■ Do exercises to increase your flexibility (see pages 48-51).

5

KYPHOSIS

An exaggerated thoracic curve that gives a hunchback appearance is known as kyphosis. It may be present at birth, but more often it is the result of adopting a bad posture over many years with the result that the back muscles become weak and over-stretched. It may also be caused by osteoporosis, so it often affects the elderly, especially women.

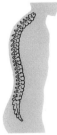

Kyphosis

COUNTERING KYPHOSIS

- Maintain good posture (see pages 68-71).

- Do back strengthening exercises daily (see pages 52-55).

- Make sure work surfaces are at the correct height (see pages 62-63).

- Avoid bending.

- Take preventive measures to counter osteoporosis (see pages 96-97).

- Learn to relax.

LORDOSIS

An excessive forward curve of the lumbar spine is known as a lordosis. Causes include: poor posture, with the bottom and chest stuck out; pregnancy, because of the weight of the baby in the abdomen; weak abdominal muscles; obesity; and osteoarthritis of the hip – this tends to make the chest lean forward and the bottom stick out.

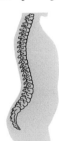

Lordosis

COUNTERING LORDOSIS

- Maintain good posture (see pages 68-71), especially during pregnancy.

- Do back and stomach strengthening exercises (see pages 52-55) daily.

ANKYLOSING SPONDYLITIS

Ankylosing spondylitis is a rheumatic, degenerative disease that runs in families and mainly affects young men between the ages of 20 and 40; women are affected, too, but to a lesser degree. The first sign of the disease is low back pain and stiffness in the morning. As it progresses up to the neck, the joints of the vertebral column become fused together, and the disks and ligaments harden until the spine forms a rigid bow. At this stage, the condition is sometimes called "bamboo spine." Ankylosing spondylitis is a serious condition that requires medical treatment: normally this consists of exercise, physical therapy, and anti-inflammatory drugs, all of which are intended to keep the spine supple for as long as possible. Pain is not always continuous, but radiotherapy may be used in cases when it is severe.

5

NON-SPINAL BACK PAIN

Back pain is not always caused by a problem in the back. Pain in other areas of the body can "refer" pain to the spinal region – sometimes this is because two areas of the body share the same pain pathways. A number of general illnesses, such as flu, can also produce backache, as can conditions affecting certain internal organs.

IF IN DOUBT, SEE YOUR DOCTOR

If your pain is not altered by movement or a change in position, then it is possible its cause is not spinal and you should consult your doctor. The panel below lists some of the non-spinal conditions that can cause back pain.

MEDICAL CAUSES OF BACK PAIN

Gynecological problems	■ Premenstrual syndrome and menstrual cramps are often felt as a dull pain in the lower back.
	■ Inflammation or infection of the female reproductive organs produces back pain, normally with abdominal pain.
Abdominal problems	■ An inflamed pancreas can cause a deep pain in the mid-back – this may be due to excessive alcohol intake.
	■ Inflammation of the gallbladder or gallstones produces pain under one or both shoulder blades accompanied by stomach cramps and nausea.
	■ Kidney infections and kidney stones can cause severe pain in the lower back, often with nausea.
	■ Stomach ulcers can cause a pain in the mid-back, especially after meals.
Chest problems	■ Heart problems may give rise to pain in the mid-back, usually with severe chest pains.
	■ A lung infection may cause pain in the mid-back. It is usually accompanied by chest pain and feverishness.
General problems	■ Influenza causes a generalized backache as well as a high temperature.
	■ Meningitis causes severe neck pain and stiffness as well as a high temperature.
	■ A benign or malignant tumor.

5

PROFESSIONAL HELP

Sometimes a back problem fails to respond to the short-term self-help remedies of rest and exercise, or to longer term measures, such as posture correction and weight loss. In such cases, it is important to consult your doctor. This is not only to rule out any underlying disorder but to take advantage of a range of treatments that your doctor can recommend for you. In serious cases, it may be necessary to see a specialist and undergo tests and, sometimes, surgery – though this is very much the last resort. However, physical therapy, osteopathy, chiropractic, acupuncture, and the Alexander Technique can all be effective forms of treatment. This chapter describes the professional options that might be of help to you.

PHYSICAL THERAPY

The most common first choice of treatment for back problems is physical therapy. This therapy uses physical methods, either alone or as an adjunct to drugs or surgery, in treatment: manipulative techniques, exercises, hydrotherapy, and heat, cold, or electrical treatments, as well as correcting posture and advising on how to carry out daily activities. Physical therapists can only practice if they are registered as qualified to do so by the health authorities, having qualified after an extensive course of study and training.

HYDROTHERAPY

Most hospital physical therapy departments have a hydrotherapy pool that people with back complaints can use, under supervision, as part of their physical therapy treatment. However, in some countries – Austria, Germany, and Switzerland, in particular – hydrotherapy is one of the main forms of treatment for a number of conditions, including back problems. Hydrotherapy is particularly useful when treating these, because water supports the body, taking most of its weight so muscles can move freely without straining to maintain a position. This means that joints that are normally weight-bearing, such as those in the spine, can be put through their full range of movements without being squashed together. Swimming, especially in a warm pool, is also a good way of easing muscle spasms and tension, building up weak muscles, and reducing joint stiffness. The stroke that you should use depends on the nature of your back problem:

■ Backstroke is particularly beneficial for those with rounded shoulders and kyphosis (page 101), and helps to strengthen stomach muscles.

■ The crawl eases muscle spasms in the upper back and strengthens the spinal muscles.

■ Breaststroke should be avoided if you have low back pain as the stroke tends to make the lumbar spine arch too much and an unequal leg kick puts strain on the lumbar joints.

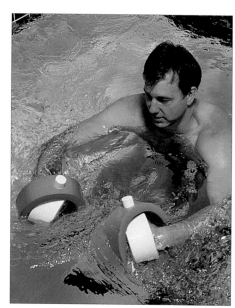

Exercise in warm water, which supports the body's weight, eases muscle spasm and tension and improves mobility.

6

THE RANGE OF TREATMENTS

Both acute and chronic back problems often react well to a course of physical therapy. Specific treatments depend on the nature of the problem, but they may include:

Manipulation and mobilization	Gentle repetitive movements restore the full range of movement and ease muscle spasm.
Heat treatment	Heat lamps warm the skin and superficial tissues to ease tension and muscle spasm; short-wave and microwave diathermy heat the deep tissues by means of electromagnetic waves to relieve pain and reduce muscle spasm and stiffness.
Cold treatment	Cold packs combat muscle spasms and reduce any bruising or swelling.
Hydrotherapy	See facing page.
Ultrasound treatment	An ultrasound machine emits high-frequency sound waves that are inaudible to the human ear. The waves penetrate through the skin and help to relax muscles, reduce swelling, and relieve pain. They also promote healing of tissues but have no effect on bones.
Traction	The spine is stretched longitudinally, either manually or with the help of special equipment. This often relieves pain and aids relaxation.
Exercises	Three types of exercise are used. In passive exercises the physical therapist moves the joints through their full range of movement to ease joint congestion and swelling, relieve tension, and promote mobility. Isometric exercises are used when movement produces pain and muscle spasm. The patient contracts the appropriate muscles without causing any movement, holds the contraction for a few seconds, and then relaxes. Active exercise is the most frequently used type for a bad back. The patient is given graded exercises that are initially performed under the supervision of the physical therapist.

ALTERNATIVE THERAPIES

Conventional medicine is not always successful when it comes to treating chronic conditions, such as long-term back pain. In such cases, it is worth considering one of the alternative, or complementary, therapies that have a good reputation in treating cases involving back problems. However, it is important that you choose an experienced practitioner who has the appropriate training and qualifications – otherwise, you run the risk of causing more damage to your back. If you are considering trying one of these therapies for your back problem, it is best to discuss the advisability of this type of treatment with your doctor first. Some back conditions should not be treated in this way (see box).

OSTEOPATHY

Osteopathy was devised by Andrew Taylor Still, an American engineer and medical doctor, in the late 19th century. He looked at the human body as a machine and believed that many ailments were the result of a misalignment in the bones, muscles, and ligaments of the body that put undue stress on the body. As a result, the aim of osteopathy is to align the body correctly, so reducing muscular tension and increasing joint flexibility. Trials have shown that osteopathic treatment can be very successful in the treatment of back problems. Osteopathy treatments include:

■ Massage: deep kneading, trigger point massage, and localized massage.

■ Passive stretching of muscles and joints.

■ Manipulation: both localized thrusts and indirect pulls.

CHIROPRACTIC

At around the same time that Andrew Still was developing osteopathy, Daniel Palmer, a Canadian working in Iowa, devised a therapy he named chiropractic. Palmer believed that the back, with its extensive nervous and musculoskeletal system, was the source of many ailments. He discovered that manipulating the spine into a correct alignment improved nerve function and benefitted many other areas and functions of the body. Chiropractors have a repertoire of more than 100 different manipulations from which to choose, depending on the treatment that is needed. Research shows that chiropractic treatment performed by a qualified practitioner benefits many patients with back problems, both in the short and long term. Chiropractic treatments include:

■ Manipulation, including short localized thrusts and "lever pulls" that twist the entire body.

■ Localized ice treatment to reduce swelling and relieve pain.

6

ACUPUNCTURE, ACUPRESSURE, AND SHIATSU

A 1973 study by The Royal Society of Medicine in Britain found that nine out of ten people suffering from muscular aches and pains showed some improvement after treatment with acupuncture. This ancient Chinese therapy is based on the belief that the

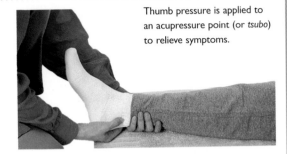

Thumb pressure is applied to an acupressure point (or *tsubo*) to relieve symptoms.

body's life force – *chi* – flows through energy channels called meridians, and that the flow can be altered beneficially by stimulating the meridians with needles at the points at which they pass close to the skin. Acupressure follows the same principle, except that variable pressure from the finger or thumb is used instead of needles, making it more of a self-help treatment. Shiatsu, a therapy that was developed in Japan, follows many of the same ideas as acupuncture and acupressure. Practitioners of shiatsu use pressure from the elbows and knees, as well as thumbs, to stimulate specific sites, known as *tsubos*.

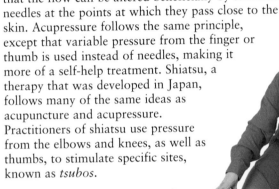

A shiatsu therapist "senses" the flow of energy between the pressure point and the area being treated.

CHECKING QUALIFICATIONS

Regulations regarding the training and registration by the health authorities of practitioners in these disciplines vary from country to country. In some countries, it is possible to advertise one's services as a practitioner without any training or qualification. If in doubt, contact a national organization representing practitioners in these areas and ask for a recommendation.

Warning

None of the above treatments should be used on somebody suffering from bone cancer, rheumatoid arthritis, or osteoporosis. If in doubt, contact your physician first.

6

ALEXANDER TECHNIQUE

In the course of life, we all tend to adopt poor habits of posture and motion, which in time come to feel "right." But these bad habits can place a large amount of unnecessary stress on the musculoskeletal system and this, in turn, can affect the smooth running of the rest of the body. The Alexander Technique is a system by which the body's posture and movement are reeducated.

THE ORIGINS OF THE TECHNIQUE

The Alexander Technique was developed by F. M. Alexander, an Australian actor born in Tasmania in the middle of the 19th century who had a problem with his voice. After doctors had failed to cure it, Alexander noticed that he often used his head in an unnatural way – he pulled it back and down while talking – and trained himself to move his head in a more balanced and natural way. The result was that the problem with his voice disappeared. After a while, Alexander gave up acting and devoted himself to developing a complete system that would rid people of "poor use" habits and promote and maintain "good use" in everyday life.

Alexander wrote four books, the most useful of which is *The Use of Self*, and started to train others to teach his system. Today Alexander teachers have to complete a three-year training course before they can be registered by the Society of Teachers of the Alexander Technique.

COMMON FAULTS

The Alexander Technique identifies a number of common faults with posture and movement:

- The whole body is slouched.
- One shoulder is held higher than the other.
- One arm is held farther forward than the other.
- The shoulders are always tense.
- The head pokes forward when walking.
- The knees are braced right back when standing.
- The knees are either allowed to roll out when sitting or are crossed.
- The head is pulled too far back and the back is bent while sitting down.
- When sitting, the feet either do not touch the ground or are bent under the chair with only the toes in contact with the ground.

RECOMMENDED FOR

- Poor posture
- Back problems
- Joint pain
- Chronic muscular tension
- Headaches
- Tiredness
- Stress
- Breathing problems
- Ankylosing spondylitis
- Osteoarthritis

6

THE TECHNIQUE IN PRACTICE

Some teachers teach groups, but most work with individual students on a one-to-one basis. A course of lessons usually consists of around ten sessions, each lasting between half an hour and an hour. Teachers use both their hands and voice commands to help students move correctly from one position to another, asking them to repeat movements until the students can "feel" the correct position and maintain it. With practice, students become aware of the correct alignment and relationship to each other of the head, neck, and back in all movements and positions. Old habits are shed, and the body begins to move freely and economically once more.

CORRECTING POSTURE THE ALEXANDER WAY

An Alexander teacher looks at the body at rest and during movement and tries to restrain bad habits and educate in new and healthier ways.

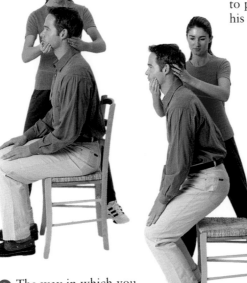

1 The teacher looks at the angle of the neck, and the way in which the neck is supported, and uses gentle pressure to prevent the pupil from pulling his head back.

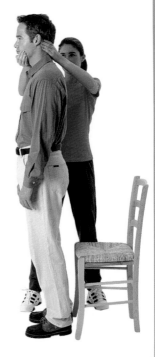

2 The way in which you move from a sitting to a standing position is a key area of concern. It is important to maintain the alignment of the neck and spine throughout the movement.

3 In the standing position, the teacher encourages a balanced upright posture before the pupil starts to walk.

6

MEDICINE AND SURGERY

If an attack of acute back pain persists without any reduction of pain after 24 hours of rest and exercise, or if you have chronic back pain, you should consult your doctor. Depending on the diagnosis, you may be given painkillers and advised to rest and exercise, referred to a physical therapist or complementary therapist, such as an osteopath, or, in more serious cases, recommended to see an orthopedic surgeon.

CONSULTING YOUR DOCTOR

Diagnosing the problem

Your doctor is likely to take a general medical history of you and your family to rule out any underlying disorder. Then you will be asked a number of questions.

- Where is the pain?
- What type of pain is it?
- What were you doing when you first felt the pain?
- How long have you had it?
- Has it moved at all?
- Is there a position in which you are pain-free?
- What type of work do you do?
- How much exercise do you do, and of what type?

Physical examination

The doctor is also likely to carry out a physical examination of your back.

- Examining the spine for any tenderness.
- Testing range of movement of the spine when standing and lying.
- Testing muscle strength.
- Noting your posture when sitting, standing still, and walking.
- Testing for any numbness.
- Testing your reflexes at the knee and at the ankles.

Treatment and referral

Depending on what the history and examination reveal, the doctor is likely to recommend further treatment at home or more extensive evaluation and testing.

- Bed rest for a few days to allow any inflammation to die down.
- Painkillers with anti-inflammatory drugs, and sometimes tranquilizers to help ease muscle spasm.
- An injection of a corticosteroid drug into the painful point – as, for example, a stubborn trigger point.
- Physical therapy or osteopathy.
- An X-ray to check for osteophyte formation, a fracture, or a misplaced vertebra.
- A corset to support the spine.
- A bone density scan to rule out osteoporosis.
- Referral to an orthopedic surgeon or neurologist.

6

SPECIALIZED TESTS

Before deciding on the appropriate course of treatment, a specialist might ask for one of the following tests to be carried out:

■ **Myelography** – a radio-opaque substance is injected into the spinal column under local anesthetic so the specialist can see whether the spinal column has become too narrow (spinal stenosis).

■ **Discography** – a radio-opaque material is injected into the vertebral disks to show whether there has been a prolapse or any shrinkage.

■ **CAT scan** (computerized-axial-tomography) – numerous X-rays are combined to provide a cross-sectional picture of the body, layer by layer, that reveals any disk damage, osteophytes, or narrowing of the spinal canal.

SURGICAL PROCEDURES

The majority of back problems are the result of poor posture, incorrect use of muscles, or soft tissue damage. As a result, surgery is the last resort in the treatment of back problems. However, the following procedures are available for cases in which other treatments have failed and the back problem is causing severe disability:

■ The injection of a corticosteroid drug combined with a painkiller into an inflamed facet joint under local anesthetic by an anesthetist.

■ **Chemonucleolysis** – this is a relatively new procedure, in which a chemical derived from the pawpaw (papaya) fruit is injected into a prolapsed disk causing it to shrink and harden. The technique is usually used in the case of young people who have not had a prolapsed disk for long, so there is no permanent nerve damage.

■ **Discectomy** – a prolapsed disk is removed under general anesthetic in order to relieve a trapped nerve root.

■ **Facetectomy** – any osteophytes or bony thickenings (stenosis) from around the spinal canal or the passages through which the spinal nerves pass are removed under general anesthetic, to free any nerve roots and widen the vertebral arch or spinal canal.

■ **Spinal fusion** – bone is taken from the hip bone and grafted across two vertebrae to fuse them and prevent any further malformation of the spine in order to stabilize it and to fix an area in which movement causes pain; sometimes wire rods and screws are used to fix the vertebrae. The patient remains on bed rest for at least a week and has to wear a corset when he or she is allowed up. This is a major operation, and complete recovery can take up to a year.

6

INDEX

A
acupuncture/acupressure 107
acute back pain 24
  causes of 22
  do's and don'ts for recovery 31
  lying on your side 30
  position for pain relief 26
  questionnaire about problems 25
  self-treatment aids 31
  see also exercises for acute back pain
acute pain 18
Alexander Technique 108
ankylosing spondylitis 101

B
back corset 34
back pain, non-spinal 102
back strain 60
  steps for avoiding 61
bathroom, and back strain 66
bed, choosing a 86
body-type and your back 81
bones 12
  and osteoarthritis 95

C
cartilage, degeneration of 95
chiropractic 106
chronic back pain 45
  and disease 41
  muscular causes 40
  relief of 44
  skeletal causes 42
  see also exercises for chronic back pain
chronic pain 18

D
desktop, working at a 75
diet 83
  and weight 82
disks 13
  shrinkage of 42
  slipped (prolapsed) 13
doctor, consulting your 110
dowager's hump 96
driving, and back strain 60

E
endorphins 20
exercise
  excessive/unaccustomed 23
  to regain mobility 36
  lack of 40
  regular 58
  warning 29
exercises for acute back pain
  immediate 27
  secondary 28
exercises for chronic back pain
  back strengthening 52
  flexibility 48
  increasing flexibility 50
  second-stage back strengthening 54
  warm-up 46
  warning 44

F, G
facet joint problems 43
fitness, general 58
  physical benefits 59
gardening, and back care 78

H, I
high heels 60
housework techniques 64
  ironing 64
  making the bed 65
  vacuuming 65
  washing 65
hydrotherapy 104
intervertebral disks see disks

K, L
kitchen
  adapting work surfaces 62
  storage 63
  washing up 63
kyphosis 101
lifting 76
  incorrect 23
  correct 77
ligaments 13
lordosis 101

M, N, O
massage 32
  warning 33
mobility, regaining
  do's and don'ts 38
  exercises 36
muscles
  abdominal 14
  back 14
  imbalance/weakness 41
neck collar 34
nerve fibers 20
  A-fibers 18
  C-fibers 18
osteoarthritis 94
osteopathy 106
osteophytes 95
osteoporosis 96
  preventing 97
over-the-counter medicines 35
overweight 80

P, R
pain 18
  gateways 19
  thresholds 19
painkillers 35
  natural 20
  overuse, and pain 45
pelvic tilt
  lying 27
  sitting/standing 57

physical therapy treatments 105
postnatal exercises 92
posture 68
  correcting by exercise 70
  good standing 69
  poor and spinal alignment 40
  poor standing 68
pregnancy, and back pain 88
  exercises in 90
referred pain 42
relaxation 84
rubbing it better 19

S
sciatica 98
  do's and don'ts 99
scoliosis 100
shiatsu 107
sitting 73
  correct seated angle 72
sleep 85
spinal cord 16
spinal nerves 17
spine
  and accidents 17
  bends in the 100
  curves of 11
  lessening pressure on 24
  structure of 10
stretches 56
  warning 56
surgical procedures 111

T, V, W
tendons 14
tests, specialist 111
trigger points 33
vertebrae 12
vertebral column, range of movement 15
weight 80
  and diet 82
  and your spine 81
workplace, back care at 74

ACKNOWLEDGMENTS

The author and the publishers gratefully acknowledge the invaluable contributions made by Paul Forrester who took all the photographs in this book except:

16 Zara McCalmont/The Garden Picture Library; 23 top Regine M/The Image Bank; bottom Bob Martin/Tony Stone Images; 58 Marc Romanelli/The Image Bank; 59 Alan Evrard/Robert Harding Picture Library; 94 The Stock Market; 97 top The Image Bank; 104 John Greim/Science Photo Library. The illustrations were produced by Janos Marffy.